RHEUMATOLOGIC
REHABILITATION SERIES

VOLUME 5
SURGICAL REHABILITATION

EDITORS
Jeanne L. Melvin
MS, OTR, FAOTA
Victoria Gall
MEd, PT

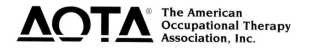

AOTA® The American
Occupational Therapy
Association, Inc.

The American Occupational Therapy Association, Inc.
4720 Montgomery Lane
PO Box 31220
Bethesda, Maryland 20824-1220

Disclaimers
This publication is designed to provide accurate and authoritative information in regard to the subject matter covered. It is sold or distributed with the understanding that the publisher is not engaged in rendering legal, accounting, or other professional service. If legal advice or other expert assistance is required, the services of a competent professional person should be sought.
—From the Declaration of Principles jointly adopted by the American Bar Association and a Committee of Publishers and Associations

It is the objective of The American Occupational Therapy Association to be a forum for free expression and interchange of ideas. The opinions expressed be the contributors to this work are their own and not necessarily those of either the editors or the American Occupational therapy Association.

ISBN 1-56900-114-6

Dedication

Clement B. Sledge, MD

A pioneer in surgery for rheumatoid arthritis, Dr. Sledge is a gifted surgeon, researcher, and educator. His research on bone and cartilage metabolism and prosthetic knee design has influenced all surgeons. His foresight to organize the Total Joint Registry has resulted in the documentation of long-term outcomes of more than 25,000 total hip and knee replacement surgeries, a critical tool for the refinement of these surgeries and for optimal patient care. Through his leadership as Chairman of the Department of Orthopedic Surgery at Brigham and Women's Hospital (Boston, MA) and earlier at the Robert B. Brigham Hospital and in numerous national and international organizations, he has championed rehabilitation and patient education. Finally, Dr. Sledge has the extraordinary ability to cut to the heart of a complex subject and express it with clarity to the benefit to all who have been fortunate enough to train and work with him or to read the books he has edited—*The Textbook of Rheumatology: Arthritis Surgery* or *Orthopedic Radiology*, including the Editors of this book.

Table of Contents

Preface to the *Rheumatologic Rehabilitation Series*

The specialty practice area of rheumatologic rehabilitation has been created in large part by the Association of Rheumatology Health Professionals (ARHP), which was founded to support interdisciplinary communication and education. The effect of the ARHP and its philosophy is manifest in the concept of this series and in the spirit of cooperation shown by the contributing authors, many of whom joined this project specifically because it is an interdisciplinary educational endeavor.

This book is the direct result of the first ARHP Fellowship (1973–1974) from the ARHP and the Arthritis Foundation, which made it possible for me to research and write *Rheumatic Disease in the Adult and Child: Occupational Therapy and Rehabilitation* (Melvin, 1977), which was published in 1977 and then continued into three editions. Although the present series was initially intended to be a revision and expansion of that textbook to include physical therapy, there is now little left of the previous text except organizational design, some illustrations, and a few paragraphs in volumes 2 and 3.

This series focuses on educating physical and occupational therapy practitioners because these two professions share knowledge bases in the areas of anatomy, physiology, rheumatology, and rehabilitation to be competent in the physical rehabilitation of persons with rheumatic diseases. Additionally, these practitioners often work together to achieve the desired outcomes for this patient population. But, of course, we hope that all professionals interested in the rehabilitation of persons with rheumatic diseases will find this series useful.

We tackle the task of educating practitioners about rheumatologic rehabilitation in an unprecedented format. First, the content is divided into five volumes so that practitioners in adult, pediatric, hand, and orthopedic practice areas can select the volumes most relevant to their interests. The theoretical and research basis for evaluation and treatment is presented in volume 1 to facilitate the use of this material in occupational therapy and physical therapy curricula. Second, all of the disease chapters in volumes 2 and 3 demonstrate the team approach because they are written collaboratively by a rheumatologist, a physical therapist, and an occupational therapist. In volume 5, *Surgical Rehabilitation*, most chapters are authored by an orthopedic surgeon, an occupational therapist, a physical therapist, and an orthopedic nurse. Third, each chapter in all of the volumes except volume 4 (on the hand) have been reviewed from both physical therapy and occupational therapy perspectives by the coeditors.

Eighty-six authors from all health professions involved in caring for persons with rheumatic diseases have contributed to this series, which testifies to the editors' commitment to training practitioners in the multidisciplinary approach to treatment. The size of this series and the number of contributing authors reflect the growth of rheumatologic rehabilitation in all of the treating disciplines (e.g., rheumatology, orthopedic surgery, nursing, patient education, psychology, social work, pedorthics). In each of these fields, research is being conducted that directly affects the practice of occupational and physical therapy. It is no longer sufficient or even possible to learn about rheumatologic rehabilitation as a specialty area in physical therapy or occupational therapy from within a single practice area. For physical therapy and occupational therapy, the new frontiers in rheumatologic rehabilitation during the next 20 years will not necessarily be in advanced interventions unique to each field but rather will be in integrating into practice the research from the areas of patient education, wellness studies, pain management, adherence research, fatigue management, and outcome and functional evaluation. In volume 1, we have invited leading researchers and clinicians from all these fields to share the latest research and methodologies that are specifically relevant to physical and occupational therapy intervention. Within the fields of physical therapy and occupational therapy, we have invited both specialists in rheumatologic rehabilitation and in evaluation or treatment outside of arthritis treatment that could broaden the approach to treatment in rheumatology.

Jeanne L. Melvin, MS, OTR, FAOTA
Program Manager, Chronic Pain and Fibromyalgia Programs
Cedars-Sinai Medical Center, Los Angeles, California

Preface to Volume 5: Surgical Rehabilitation

The first chapter of this volume, "Surgical Rehabilitation for Arthritis: Achieving Optimal Results," focuses on surgical rehabilitation for the patient with severe polyarticular rheumatic disease, the role of preoperative evaluation, and current research on preoperative education and physical conditioning in physical therapy. This is followed by six chapters that each discuss surgery and rehabilitation for a specific joint. We invited internationally recognized surgeons and practitioners from leading hospitals to share their expertise and clinical experience in providing care for the patient with severe polyarticular rheumatoid arthritis as well as monoarticular osteoarthritis: Susan Manning-Kloos, OTR, CHT, Bryan J. Nestor, MD, and Mark P. Figgie, MD, from the Hospital for Special Surgery in New York discuss elbow surgery. Thomas S. Thornhill, MD, Victoria Gall, MEd, PT, Susan Vermette, OTR, and Frances Griffin, RN, BSN, from Brigham and Women's Hospital in Boston discuss shoulder surgery. James Coyle, MD, and Rick B. Delamarter, MD, from the University of California in Los Angeles, CA, and Jeanne L. Melvin, MS, OTR, FAOTA, discuss spine surgery specifically for rheumatoid arthritis. Scott David Martin, MD, and Robert Poss, MD, from Brigham and Women's Hospital; Kathleen Zavadak, PT, and Jill Noaker, OTR, CHT, from Saint Margaret Hospital in Pittsburgh, PA; and Mary Ann Jacobs, RN, from the Jewish Hospitals of St. Louis, MO, discuss hip surgery. Thomas Sculco, MD, and Sandy B. Ganz, MS, PT, from the Hospital for Special Surgery join Jill Noaker, OTR, CHT, and Mary Ann Jacobs, RN, to discuss knee surgery. Finally, Andrea Cracchiolo, III, MD, from the University of California at Los Angeles teams up with Denise Janisse, a pedorthist (a specialist in prescription footwear and orthoses) and President of the National Pedorthic Association, and Victoria Gall, MEd, PT, to discuss foot and ankle surgery for rheumatoid arthritis. (Hand and wrist surgery is discussed in volume 4 of this series.)

Outcome evaluations of joint surgery are now conducted on the basis of function and general health status with an emphasis on patient self-report. Several of the more popular functional evaluations for the hip, knee, foot, shoulder, and elbow are featured in this volume.

Long-term outcome studies on joint arthroplasties have become a guiding force in the direction and development of orthopedic surgery. Similar studies are necessary that document the benefits of preoperative evaluation, the optimal preoperative education format, and postoperative therapy. Standards of care must be developed for specific postoperative physical therapy and occupational therapy interventions. Postoperative therapy takes place because most surgeons and practitioners believe it is essential and beneficial, not because it has been proven effective. The recent surprising research on preoperative strengthening and fitness conditioning for total hip and knee arthroplasties, reviewed in chapter 1, that demonstrates that such strengthening and conditioning do *not* improve surgical outcome emphasizes the need for research on clinical interventions.

On a personal note, Vicky Gall and I worked together from 1977 to 1980 at the Robert B. Brigham Hospital in Boston, MA, which was a 100-bed rheumatic disease hospital for Harvard Medical School under the orthopedic leadership of Clement Sledge, MD. In 1980, that hospital merged with Brigham and Women's Hospital. Vicky has worked with surgical and nonsurgical rheumatic disease patients for more than 25 years. She is one of the most knowledgeable rehabilitation clinicians in the field of rheumatologic and surgical rehabilitation. It has been a pleasure to work with Vicky again in the production of this book.

Jeanne L. Melvin, MS, OTR, FAOTA
Program Manager, Chronic Pain and Fibromyalgia Programs
Cedars-Sinai Medical Center, Los Angeles, California

Reference

Melvin, J. L. (1977). *Rheumatic disease in the adult and child: Occupational therapy and rehabilitation.* Philadelphia: F. A. Davis.

About the Authors

James Coyle, MD, is Clinical Instructor of Orthopaedic Surgery, UCLA Medical Center, Department of Orthopedics, Los Angeles, California.

Andrea Cracchiolo, III, MD, is Professor of Orthopaedic Surgery, University of California-Los Angeles, Los Angeles, California.

Rick B. Delamarter, MD, is Co-Director, University of California-Los Angeles Comprehensive Spine Center, Los Angeles, California.

Mark P. Figgie, MD, is Associate Attending of Orthopaedic Surgery, Hospital for Special Surgery, New York, New York.

Victoria Gall, M.Ed., PT, Orthopaedic and Rheumatology Services, Brigham and Women's Hospital, Boston, Massachusetts. Ms. Gall is currently in the Peace Corps in Turkmenistan.

Sandy B. Ganz, PT, MS, GCS, is Director of Rehabilitation, Amsterdam Nursing Home, and Associate in Research, Hospital for Special Surgery, New York, New York.

Frances T. Griffin, RN, BSN, is Registered Nurse, Robert B. Brigham Arthritis Center, Brigham and Women's Hospital, Boston, Massachusetts.

Mary Ann Jacobs, RN, MSN, CRRN, CS, is Rehabilitation Nurse Practitioner, Barnes-Jewish Hospital, St. Louis, Missouri.

Dennis Janisse, CPed, is CEO and President, National Pedorthic Services, Milwaukee, Wisconsin.

Susan Manning-Kloos, OTR, CHT, is a Hand Therapist, Long Island Hand Center, Huntington, New York.

Scott David Martin, MD, is Clinical Instructor in Orthopaedic Surgery, Harvard Medical School, Brigham and Women's Hospital, Boston, Massachusetts.

Jeanne L. Melvin, MS, OTR, FAOTA, is Program Manager, Chronic Pain and Fibromyalgia Programs, Cedars-Sinai Medical Center, Beverly Hills, California.

Bryan J. Nestor, MD, is Attending Surgeon, Hospital for Special Surgery, New York, New York.

Jill Noaker, OTR, CHT, is Director of Occupational Therapy, University of Pittsburgh Medical Center, St. Margaret Hospital, Pittsburgh, Pennsylvania.

Robert Poss, MD, is Professor of Orthopedic Surgery, Harvard Medical School, Brigham and Women's Hospital, Boston, Massachusetts.

Thomas P. Sculco, MD, is Director of Orthopedic Surgery, and chief, Surgical Arthritis Service, Hospital for Special Surgery, New York, New York.

Thomas S. Thornhill, MD, is Chairman, Department of Orthopedic Surgery, Harvard Medical School, Brigham and Women's Hospital, Boston, Massachusetts.

Susan Vermette, OTR, Brigham and Women's Hospital, Boston, Massachusetts.

Kathryn Haffner Zavadak, PT, was Senior Physical Therapist, Clinical Education/Rheumatology, St. Margaret Memorial Hospital, Pittsburgh, Pennsylvania, at the time of writing.

Acknowledgments

We thank all of the contributors to this volume. Collaborating on a multidisciplinary chapter required more drafts and revisions than a single-author chapter, and it required each author to make room for another's point of view. This collaboration has resulted in seven unique chapters that reflect a broad multidisciplinary view of surgery and postoperative rehabilitation. We are also indebted to the staff members at the American Occupational Therapy Association who made the series possible.

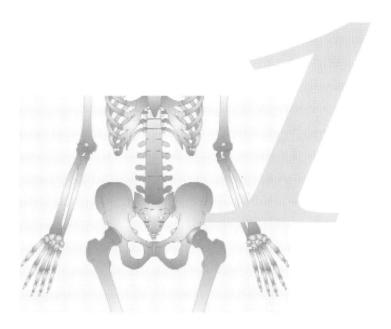

SURGICAL REHABILITATION
FOR ARTHRITIS:
ACHIEVING OPTIMAL RESULTS

Jeanne L. Melvin, MS, OTR, FAOTA, and Victoria Gall, MEd, PT

Historically, orthopedic surgery has been considered a last resort to be attempted after all else has failed or to be reserved for joints that are not functional. This is no longer true. Reconstructive surgery is now considered a part of total care for persons with chronic destructive joint disease. Consultation with an orthopedic surgeon early, before severe joint destruction occurs, allows patients more surgical options and optimal timing of both preventive and corrective surgery. Relief of pain and improved function are the primary goals of surgery for persons with rheumatic diseases, and, in selected cases, prevention of disability is the goal.

Achieving optimal outcomes after joint surgery, particularly replacement arthroplasty, requires that the patient prepare for surgery, understand the postoperative precautions and limitations, and actively participate in postoperative rehabilitation (Ganz & Viellion, 1996; Jones & Blackburn, 1998).

The practitioner's role in orthopedic surgery is (a) to understand fully the surgical procedure and postoperative medical, surgical, nursing, and rehabilitation management as well clearly understand the role of other team members and the importance of coordinating and communicating with them; (b) to be aware of the signs and symptoms of postoperative complications and to report them promptly; and (c) to respect patients as members of the team and encourage their active participation throughout the postoperative phase.

Surgical Rehabilitation of the Patient With Severe Rheumatoid Arthritis

Patients with severe polyarticular rheumatoid arthritis (RA) pose different risks and challenges to rehabilitation professionals than patients with traumatic orthopedic problems or even patients with osteoarthritis (OA) who require a single surgery. Risk factors for the patient with severe RA can include: generalized weakness; poor endurance; poor gait secondary to weakness; limited range of motion (ROM); pain and instability; multiple joint deformities; compromised immune systems secondary to steroids and other medications; upper-extremity pain; instability and deformity in the shoulder, elbow, or hand that limits ambulation with aids; and extra-articular RA involvement (e.g., lungs, heart, vasculitis). Patients who receive disability payments or have limited finances may not have supportive footwear, may lack proper nutrition, may not have chairs at an appropriate height to use at home, may live in a dangerous neighborhood where community ambulation is not an option, and may have limited transportation to a therapy clinic (Morgan, Anderson, Hood, Matthews, Lee, & Alarcon 1997; Siegel, 1995) (Table 1).

Practitioners treating patients with rheumatic diseases should be familiar with comprehensive rehabilitation for the specific disease as well as rehabilitation for the specific procedure. Practitioners who evaluate a patient with ankylosing spondylitis, RA, systemic lupus erythematosus, or other

Table 1. Surgical Rehabilitation (Polyarticular Rheumatoid Arthritis vs. Monoarticular Arthritis)

Chronic Disease	Limited Disease
• Polyarticular and systemic • Nonsurgical joints need joint protection • Patient education necessary for rheumatic disease in addition to postsurgical rehabilitation • Greater need for assistive devices	• Monoarticular and nonsystemic • Not applicable • Only postsurgical rehabilitation

Table 2. Role of Occupational Therapy and Physical Therapy in Surgical Rehabilitation

Preoperative	Postoperative (Acute Care and Rehabilitation)
• Evaluation • Education • Gait training for lower-extremity surgeries • Adaptive strategies • Discharge planning	• Positioning • Orthotic fabrication and fitting • Exercise • Edema reduction • Instruction in safety precautions • Ambulation training • Joint protection training • Activities of daily living training

rheumatic diseases are in a position to recommend additional rehabilitation measures for the primary disease (Table 2).

For many patients, joint replacement surgery will improve function sufficiently for them to participate in a community exercise program, possibly for the first time. Because patients with RA may need multiple surgeries, improving physical fitness has the potential of preventing additional surgeries. Evaluation of patients' self-management skills and educating them about the options available to help them improve function, including the roles of exercise (Minor, 1998), stress management, sleep, and nutrition, can be invaluable in helping to control disease and improve health (Boutaugh & Brady, 1998). Knowledge of community resources for exercise and arthritis education is likewise extremely helpful. Practitioners who are not familiar with community resources may contact the local or state chapter of the Arthritis Foundation for a list of resources and information to give patients (see appendix at the end of the book). *Arthritis Today* magazine is an excellent resource on self-management methods, and a subscription to the publication is included with a basic membership in the Arthritis Foundation. Local community organizations and exercise facilities may offer special programs for persons with physical limitations. The Easter Seals Society offers exercise programs, both water and land based, for anyone with a physical disability. Haralson-Ferrell (1998) reviewed the wide range of local and national

Table 3. Preoperative Considerations

Age
Diagnosis (primary and secondary)
Overall health status
Pain
Functional limitations
Social role
Occupational needs and expectations
Ability to comply with postoperative rehabilitation
Medications
Family support
Living situation
Lifestyle
Discharge plan

resources available for persons with arthritis. The effect of surgery on nonsurgical joints is a major consideration, especially for patients with severe polyarticular disease. Upper-extremity immobilization for surgery as well as use of ambulation aids can result in excessive strain on the contralateral hand. Specific splints, adaptive methods, and joint protection techniques may be necessary to prevent damage to the nonsurgical hand. New methods for bed mobility may stress involved nonsurgical joints. Patients with severe upper-extremity involvement may not be able to use a trapeze or bed ladder. These devices should not be routinely used until the patient's ability to use them is observed.

Postoperative positioning in an unfamiliar bed where the patient is attached to tubes and devices that may limit motion may likewise aggravate nonsurgical joints. Reduction of nonsteroidal anti-inflammatory drugs (NSAIDs) may result in increased inflammation. Patients taking corticosteroids may have the drug increased just before surgery. Postoperative analgesics may mask pain from increased inflammation. Evaluation of the nonsurgical joints regarding the need for acute intervention will most likely be completed by nursing staff members in the acute setting but would be the practitioner's role in a rehabilitation unit or in home health care.

Even patients who have had RA for years may benefit from a review of basic education regarding joint anatomy and inflammation. This may need to be done in the rehabilitation facility or in a home health care setting. The practitioner must be familiar with the functional outcomes of joint replacement surgery to answer patients' questions on activity progression after the healing process and therapy are completed.

Preoperative Therapy Evaluation

A preoperative evaluation for lower-extremity surgeries includes the following: an evaluation of gait, ROM of the surgical joint and screening of all joints, and functional strength of all extremities and a functional evaluation. For upper-extremity surgeries, an evaluation should include ROM, strength, and function of the surgical joint and a screen of all upper-extremity joints; function of the contralateral extremity and how unilateral functioning will affect that extremity; and a functional evaluation (Table 3).

Outcome evaluations such as the SF-36 (see Appendix at the end of the book) or other quality-of-life evaluations are best done in the surgeon's office where follow-up data can be collected. Functional evaluations unique to each joint are included in the topic chapters.

The practitioner can determine how realistic the patient's expectations are and how much education is needed by asking the following questions:

- How do you feel about having the surgery?
- What do you hope it will do for you?
- How long do you expect the recovery to take?
- How much help do you think you will need after discharge home?

Discharge planning and needs evaluation after discharge are likewise part of the preoperative evaluation.

Discharge Planning

The surgeon must provide the patient with a clear picture of the length of hospitalization, the patient's postoperative functional limitations, the approximate length of recuperation, and the possible options for postoperative rehabilitation (e.g., subacute, skilled nursing, inpatient rehabilitation, home health care). Discharge planning should begin in the surgeon's office with the decision to have surgery. Arrangements for postoperative care should be made before the patient is admitted to the hospital. Evaluation of discharge plans then becomes a part of the preoperative evaluation. Many hospitals have care coordinators who are responsible for discharge planning. The planning is the same for all joint surgeries and includes support available for meal preparation, bathing, dressing, shopping, running errands, child care, and transportation. The home environment must be evaluated regarding ambulation safety, stairs, bathroom accessibility, and chair and bed adjustments for postoperative precautions (Ganz & Viellion, 1996). Some hospitals conduct home evaluations before admission. Other hospitals have created their own home therapy divisions or contract with a specific agency to facilitate coordination and quality of care. The ability to transfer in and out of a car must be addressed. Sport utility vehicles may pose as much of a problem as low sports cars. Patients must have transportation that allows them to observe postoperative precautions.

Lefebvre and Semanik (1995) recommended using open-ended questions that encourage patients to talk about their situation in their own words, such as:

- Tell me about the kind of place you live in.
- Do you feel safe there?
- Do you anticipate any problems when you return home?
- How have your family members and friends reacted to you being in the hospital?
- What kind of help have you had from friends or family members before?
- How are you spending your days now? Please describe your daily routine.
- What kinds of things frighten you about going home after the surgery?

Preoperative Education

The goal of preoperative planning is to optimize the health of the patient (Siegel, 1995). The value and purpose of preoperative education varies on the basis of the surgery, the patient, the type of education, and the surgeon. Preoperative education may differ depending on whether the patient is having surgery to restore function or to relieve pain. A patient unable to raise his or her arm or straighten an elbow or bear weight on a knee may view surgery with greater hope and confidence. The patient who can still walk despite a painful knee may be less sure of a decision to have surgery and may need far more education to understand and be confident about the process (Table 4).

Thus far, only formal preoperative education programs have been described in the literature for patients having total hip (THA) and knee (TKA) arthroplasties. These are the most frequent total joint surgeries. Total elbow, shoulder, and ankle arthroplasties occur so infrequently compared with THA and TKA that creating education groups would not be feasible, but certainly formal individual, videotape, or computer education programs could be created for these patients.

There is no question that preoperative education and planning are beneficial. In numerous studies on THA and TKA, these procedures have been shown to decrease length of stay, reduce cost, improve patient satisfaction, decrease anxiety, increase knowledge retention, improve patient cooperation with postoperative rehabilitation, improve discharge planning, and minimize complications (Butler, Hurley, Buchanan, & Smith-VanHorne, 1996; Daltroy, Morlino, Eaton, Poss, & Liang, in press; Graziano, Aronson, & Becerra, 1995; Haines & Viellion, 1990; Lichtenstein, Semaan, & Marmar, 1993; Orr, 1990; Roach, Tremblay, & Bowers, 1995; Santavirta, Lillqvist, Sarvimaki, Honkaneu, Konttinen, & Santavirt, 1994).

The content and method of education varies. The Hospital for Special Surgery (New York, NY) created a preoperative education program for patients with a THA or TKA that consisted of education, physical therapy evaluation, and psychosocial evaluation. A 90-min educational session is

Table 4. Preoperative Education Topics

Joint anatomy
Disease process specific to the surgical joint
Surgical procedure
Length of hospitalization
Risks and benefits
Long-term results
Precautions and rationales
Postoperative positioning, skin care, equipment, and adaptive strategies
Pain management
Postoperative physical therapy and occupational therapy
Preparations for hospitalization
Proper footwear for safe ambulation
Preparations for discharge
Preventing infections
Questions and answers

presented by the physical therapist, nurse, and social worker 2 weeks before surgery. The session includes an educational booklet on facilitating recovery prepared by staff members. Analysis of functional milestones and length of stay showed that patients with THA who participated in the education program were able to ambulate with a cane and negotiate stairs unassisted 1.6 days earlier than those who did not attend. Their length of stay was shortened for the following procedures: unilateral THA, 1.5 days; bilateral THA, 1.2 days; THA revisions, 3.4 days; unilateral TKA, 0.7 days; and bilateral TKA, 4.8 days. Patient satisfaction with the program and recovery time was quite high (Graziano et al., 1995).

Wellesley Hospital (Toronto, Ontario, Canada) has a preadmission education program for patients with THA and TKA in which patients are shown a videotape explaining the procedure that includes postoperative patients getting out of a shower, dressing, and walking with crutches. This videotape provides modeling and gives patients hope that they will be able to function immediately after the surgery. Patients are additionally given a booklet on how to prepare for the hospital and some basic exercises.

The Arthritis Society of Canada offers monthly educational classes to persons considering hip or knee surgery. The 90-min classes discuss anatomy of the joint, the disease process, conservative treatment principles, indications for surgery, surgical procedures, risks and benefits, postoperative strategies, and long-term results, with questions-and-answer periods included. Patients needing additional information are assisted on an individual basis (*Arthritis News*, 1995).

Daltroy, Morilino, Eaton, Pass, & Liang (in press) compared the effectiveness of a preoperative 12-min slide and videotape education program with training in Benson's Relaxation Response by using a bedside audiotape. The educational intervention reduced length of stay and pain medication use for patients who exhibited the most denial (i.e., a tendency to avoid thinking about unpleasant events) and reduced postoperative anxiety and cognitive errors on the Mini-Mental State Exam for patients with the most baseline anxiety. Education did not have an effect on postoperative pain. The Benson Relaxation Response did not influence postoperative outcomes. (This occurred in part because the patients did not have enough time to practice the technique.) High preoperative anxiety was associated with greater postoperative anxiety, pain and use of analgesic medication, poorer mental status, and longer stays in the hospital.

Preoperative Physical Conditioning

For years, there has been a question regarding whether preoperative physical conditioning makes a difference in the postoperative outcome of THA and TKA. There are now three controlled studies that have examined this issue and were unable to demonstrate any notable difference in patients receiving several weeks of formal preoperative conditioning in physical therapy compared with patients receiving no preoperative conditioning. Weidenhielm, Mattson, Brostrom, Lars-Ake, and Wersall-Robertson (1993) in Sweden evaluated the effectiveness of 5 weeks of physical therapy on improving ROM and strength, 3 times a week, combined with a daily home program of knee ROM and lower-extremity strengthening exercises on patients with OA scheduled for a unicompartmental arthroplasty. Compared with matched patients ($n=20$) who did not receive any conditioning exercise, the treated group ($n=19$) had slightly less pain and improved joint stability, walking speed, and endurance; however, their muscle strength was not improved. There was no difference in the two groups after 3 months. In fact, the treated group had lost some strength. The evaluative parameters were pain, ROM, stability, and walking capacity. Wijgman, Dekkers, Waltje, Krekels, and Arens (1994) in the Netherlands evaluated the effectiveness of preoperative strengthening and ROM exercise in physical therapy on patients with OA scheduled to have a THA compared with no preoperative intervention. The Harris Hip Score demonstrated a positive difference that favored the treated group on postoperative day 14 and at discharge. A visual analog scale and functional milestones did not indicate a difference. D'Lima, Colwell, Morris, Harwick, and Kozin (1996) at the Scripps Clinic in LaJolla, CA, examined the effect of both cardiovascular conditioning (group 3), a ROM and knee-strengthening program (group 2), and no preoperative therapy (group 1) on patients scheduled for a TKA. There were 30 patients in the study; 5 had RA, and the remainder had OA. There was no difference between the three groups postoperatively when using the Hospital for Special Surgery Knee Rating, the Arthritis Impact Measurement Scale, and the Quality of Well Being instrument. The researchers believed that the dramatic improvement from surgery and deconditioning from surgery overshadowed the small benefit seen from preoperative conditioning.

These studies may indicate that the patients were appropriate candidates for surgery in that they had such severe pain or structural damage that they were not candidates for conservative treatment. This information essentially applies to patients with OA and cannot be extrapolated to patients with RA or other polyarticular diseases who may benefit from upper- and lower-extremity strengthening to improve postoperative ambulation capacity.

Pain Management

Postoperative pain management is essential for patients to fully participate in therapy. The timing of analgesic medications should allow optimal pain relief during therapy. The reduction of anxiety through preoperative education is not a small issue because anxiety and fear can amplify pain. In the acute setting, any measures that are calming and supportive to the patient and reduce anxiety and stress can reduce pain. For the anxious patient, this could include deep breathing and training in conscious relaxation.

The continuous passive motion (CPM) machine can reduce postoperative pain. Patients report that they like having control over the device and the gentle, gradual progression of exercise. Epidural analgesics likewise have greatly reduced pain after knee surgery.

Ice is generally preferred to reduce pain and swelling on the surgical joint and is often used after therapy. Albrecht and colleagues (1997) in Germany compared the analgesic effect of a closed, continuous, cooling system that uses pumps to enable water-free cooling of the operating area with traditional intermittent cold packs of microcrystalline silicate on 312 patients after THA or TKA. Continuous cryotherapy resulted in a depression of skin temperature to 12C, whereas intermittent cooling only caused a mean temperature decrease of 1C. Clinically continuous cold application led to a more than 50% decrease of analgesic demands in both systemic and regional applications ($p < 0.001$). This significantly correlated with patient pain sensation as well as ROM. Intermittent cold packs were found to be ineffective in comparison. Many commercial cold packs are ineffective; clinicians must evaluate the effectiveness of their cold application method.

Reinforcing proper use of medications can help control pain. Many patients are fearful that they will become addicted to narcotic analgesics. Generally, patients without an addiction history and who do not like to take medications do not have a problem with dependency on postoperative narcotics.

Clinical or Critical Pathways

Clinical pathways with multidisciplinary documentation forms have proven to be an effective tool for coordinating care and communication among treating staff members. These pathways encourage staff members to support and reinforce team goals and were developed to standardize quality care. In some hospitals, clinical pathways have resulted in a reduction of length of stay and treatment costs and improved quality of care (Mukland, Fitzsimmons, Libby, Mahoney, & Zielinski, 1997; Munin, Kwoh, Glynn, Crossett, & Rubash, 1995; Thomas, Miller, Silaj, & King, 1994).

Clinical pathways can be developed for the patient and family members so that they can understand the progression of care. An example of this is the patient and family member critical care pathway for THA and TKA used at Brigham and Women's Hospital in Boston (See appendices in chapters 5 and 6).

Surgical Timing

To encourage appropriate patient motivation for surgery, orthopedic surgeons generally do not try to convince patients to have surgery. Surgeons explain the options, risks, and gains and require that the patient make the decision. If a patient waits until the joint is so painful that he or she "can no longer stand it," surgery is often viewed as a positive experience; the patient looks forward to a life without debilitating pain. A patient "talked into" surgery when he or she has only moderate pain may view the pain and stress of surgery with less enthusiasm. Sometimes this process encourages patients to wait too long for surgery, and the destruction from the disease becomes so severe that it makes rehabilitation more difficult.

A question that often arises is, "How early should surgery be performed?" Although the specific timing is different for each surgery, most surgeons agree that surgery should be performed only after all conservative measures have been given a fair trial and the patient is stabilized on a medication regimen. Patients who have persistent synovitis and pain for 3 to 6 months, despite conservative measures, are considered possible candidates for joint surgery (Sledge, 1993). In a traditional sense, appropriate conservative treatment for RA includes adequate trials of both NSAIDs and disease-modifying drugs, intra-articular corticosteroid injections, orthoses, thermal modalities, exercise, and joint protection training. From a holistic perspective, conservative management now includes effective self-management training that includes developing a positive psychological and emotional approach for working with illness, nutrition for optimal health, physical fitness training, and relaxation or stress management processes for improving the immune system and overall health. On the other hand, surgery for a painful, destroyed joint may enable a person to participate in fitness programs that will help their overall health.

Future Research

Standardized outcome evaluations will provide essential information on the benefits and limitations of joint surgery. These evaluations will be useful tools for investigating postoperative rehabilitation techniques such as biking, use of various ambulatory devices, types of exercise, and immobilization such casting for foot procedures and splinting for elbow arthroplasties.

Krebs and Neumann are physical therapy researchers who have expanded the knowledge base for postoperative rehabilitation with their research on hip joint pressure and biomechanics during gait. Their work should be continued and expanded to include all joints and all procedures (Krebs, Elbaum, Riley, Hodge, & Mann, 1991; Neumann, 1996; Tackson, Krebs, & Harris, 1997).

Each facility should have practice standards for all interventions that are done on a routine basis whether for quadriceps strengthening or for use of pulleys. There should be a forum for discussing and reviewing procedures and clinical pathways. The Annual Scientific Meeting of the Association of Rheumatology Health Professionals provides an opportunity for this type of multidisciplinary communication. (Information about this meeting is available on the American College of Rheumatology website: www.rheumatology.org).

References

Albrecht, S., le Blond, R., Kohler, V., Cordis, R., Gill, C., Kleihues, H., Schluter, S., & Noack, W. (1997). [Cryotherapy as analgesic technique in direct, post-operative treatment following elective joint replacement]. *Zeitschrift Fur Orthopadie Und Ihre Grenzgebiete* (Stuttgart), *135*(1), 45–51.

Arthritis and orthopaedic surgery [special issue]. (1995). *Arthritis News, 13*.

Boutaugh, M. L., & Brady, T. J. (1998). Patient education for self-management. In J. L. Melvin & G. Jensen (Eds.), *Rheumatologic rehabilitation series. Volume 1: Assessment and management* (pp. 219–258). Bethesda, MD: American Occupational Therapy Association.

Butler, G. S., Hurley, C. A., Buchanan, K. L., & Smith-VanHorne, J. (1996). Prehospital education: Effectiveness with total hip replacement surgery patients. *Patient Education and Counseling, 29*(2), 189–197.

Daltroy, L. H., Morlino, C. I., Eaton, H. M., Poss, R., & Liang, M. H. (in press). Preoperative education for total hip and knee replacement patients. *Arthritis Care and Research.*

D'Lima, D. D., Colwell, C. W. Jr., Morris, B. A., Harwick, M. E., & Kozin, F. (1996). The effect of preoperative exercise on total knee replacement outcomes. *Clinical Orthopaedics and Related Research, 326*, 174–182.

Ganz, S. B., & Viellion, G. (1996). Pre and post surgical management of the hip and knee. In S. T. Wegener (Ed.), *Clinical care in the rheumatic diseases*. Atlanta, GA: American College of Rheumatology.

Graziano, S., Aronson, S., & Becerra, J. (1995). A multidisciplinary preoperative arthroplasty education program [abstract]. *Arthritis and Rheumatism, 38*(9), S154.

Haines, N., & Viellion, G. (1990). A successful combination: Preadmission testing and preoperative education. *Orthopaedic Nursing, 9*, 53–59.

Haralson-Ferrell, K. M. (1998). Community resources in comprehensive rehabilitation. In J. Melvin & G. Jensen (Eds.), *Rheumatologic rehabilitation series. Volume 1: Assessment and management* (pp. 393–408). Bethesda, MD: American Occupational Therapy Association.

Jones, R. E., & Blackburn, W. D. Jr. (1998). Joint replacement surgery preoperative management. *Bulletin on the Rheumatic Diseases, 47*(4), 5–8.

Krebs, D. E., Elbaum, L., Riley, P. O., Hodge, W. A., & Mann, R. W. (1991). Exercise and gait effects on in vivo hip contact pressures. *Physical Therapy, 71*, 301–309.

Lefebvre, K., & Semanik, P. (1995, October). *An interview outline to assess psychosocial factors that will influence outcome in an orthopedic population.* Paper presented at the American College of Rheumatology Scientific Meeting, San Francisco, CA.

Lichtenstein, R., Semaan, S., & Marmar, E. C. (1993). Development and impact of a hospital-based perioperative patient education program in a joint replacement center. *Orthopaedic Nursing, 12*(6), 17–25.

Minor, M. A. (1998). Exercise for health and fitness. In J. L. Melvin & G. Jensen (Eds.), *Rheumatologic rehabilitation series. Volume 1: Assessment and management* (pp. 351–367). Bethesda, MD: American Occupational Therapy Association.

Morgan, S. L., Anderson, A. M., Hood, A. M., Matthews, P. A., Lee, J. Y., & Alarcon, S. G. (1997). Nutrient intake patterns, body mass index, and vitamin levels in patients with rheumatoid arthritis. *Arthritis Care and Research, 10*(1), 9–17.

Mukland, J., Fitzsimmons, C., Libby, L., Mahoney, A., & Zielinski, A. (1997, August). Critical pathways for TKR: Protocol saves time and money. *Advance for Directors in Rehabiliation,* 31–33.

Munin, M. C., Kwoh, C. K., Glynn, N., Crossett, L., & Rubash, H. E. (1995). Predicting discharge outcome after elective hip and knee arthroplasty. *American Journal of Physical Medicine and Rehabilitation, 74*(4), 294–301.

Neumann, D. A. (1996). Hip abductor muscle activity in persons with a hip prosthesis while carrying loads in one hand. *Physical Therapy, 76*, 1320–1330.

Orr, P. M. (1990). An educational program for total hip and knee replacement patients as part of a total arthritis center program. *Orthopaedic Nursing, 9*(5), 61–69.

Roach, J. A., Tremblay, L. M., & Bowers, D. L. (1995). A preoperative assessment and education program: Implementation and outcomes. *Patient Education Counseling, 25*(1), 83–88.

Santavirta, N., Lillqvist, G., Sarvimaki, A., Honkanen, V., Konttinen, Y. T., & Santavirta, S. (1994). Teaching of patients undergoing total hip replacement surgery. *International Journal of Nursing Studies, 31*(2), 135–142.

Siegel, M. B. (1995). Preparing the complicated rheumatology client for revision of a total hip arthroplasty [abstract]. *Arthritis and Rheumatism, 38*(9), S229.

Sledge, C. B. (1993). Introduction to surgical management. In W. N. Kelly, E. D. Harris, S. Ruddy, & C. B. Sledge (Eds.), *Textbook of rheumatology* (4th ed., pp. 1745–1751). Philadelphia: Saunders.

Tackson, S. J., Krebs, D. E., & Harris, B. A. (1997). Acetabular pressures during hip arthritis exercises. *Arthritis Care and Research, 10*(5), 308–319.

Thomas, J., Miller, P., Silaj, A., & King, M. L. (1994). Application of physiotherapy outcome measures to the managed care model. *Physiotherapy Canada, 46*(4), 260–265.

Weidenhielm, L., Mattsson, E., Brostrom, L. A., & Wersall-Robertsson, E. (1993). Effect of preoperative physiotherapy in unicompartmental prosthetic knee replacement. *Scandinavian Journal of Rehabilitation Medicine, 25*, 33–39.

Wijgman, A. J., Dekkers, G. H., Waltje, E., Krekels, T., & Arens, H. J. (1994). [No positive effect of preoperative exercise therapy and teaching in patient to be subjected to hip arthroplasty]. *Ned Tijdschr Geneeskd, 138*(19), 949–952.

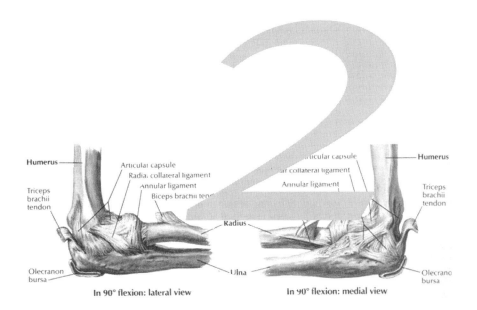

Humerus
Articular capsule
Radial collateral ligament
Annular ligament
Biceps brachii tendon
Triceps brachii tendon
Radius
Olecranon bursa
Ulna

In 90° flexion: lateral view

Articular capsule
Collateral ligament
Annular ligament
Humerus
Triceps brachii tendon
Olecranon bursa

In 90° flexion: medial view

ELBOW SURGERY AND REHABILITATION

Susan Manning-Kloos, OTR, CHT, Bryan J. Nestor, MD, and Mark P. Figgie, MD

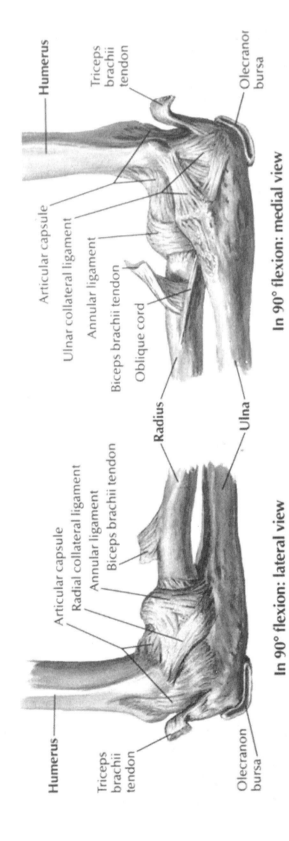

In 90° flexion: medial view

Humerus

Triceps brachii tendon

Olecranon bursa

Articular capsule

Ulnar collateral ligament

Annular ligament

Biceps brachii tendon

Oblique cord

Radius

Ulna

In 90° flexion: lateral view

Humerus

Triceps brachii tendon

Olecranon bursa

Articular capsule

Radial collateral ligament

Annular ligament

Biceps brachii tendon

Anatomy of the elbow—lateral and medial views. Copyright 1989. Novartis. Reprinted with permission from the *Atlas of Human Anatomy*, illustrated by Frank H. Netter, MD. All rights reserved.

The elbow joint is most frequently damaged by rheumatoid arthritis (RA), osteoarthritis (OA), juvenile rheumatoid arthritis (JRA), and trauma. On a less frequent basis, the elbow joint is affected by psoriatic arthritis, systemic lupus erythematosus, seronegative spondylarthropathies, infectious arthritis, crystalline arthropathies, traumatic arthritis, and tumors. Most forms of arthritis in the elbow are managed conservatively. By the time the condition is severe enough to warrant surgery, there is usually considerable disability. RA is the most common disease to cause severe pain, limited motion, and instability in the elbow. This is typically a bilateral disease, and patients who have limitations in both elbows have an added impetus to take on the risks of surgery to improve function. Many of the patients who need surgery, such as a total elbow arthroplasty (TEA), have severe polyarticular disease such as RA, and the staging of elbow surgery must be prioritized with knee, foot, and hand surgery.

Morrey, Askew, An, and Chao (1981) have shown that healthy persons use a 100° arc of motion from 30° to 130° in performing most activities of daily living (ADL). A person who has active elbow flexion of less than 90° will experience major functional limitations. Pain and loss of flexion may interfere with basic self-care, including feeding, grooming, and personal hygiene; loss of extension may interfere with lower-extremity dressing, ability to push off of a chair and desk, or work activities. Compensatory motions at the wrist, shoulder, neck, hips, and knees are often used when a healthy person has monoarticular limitation of the elbow. The patient with polyarticular arthritis is less able to compensate for lack of elbow motion than a person with monoarticular arthritis and normal proximal and distal joint mobility. Therefore, the primary goal of treatment for the patient with elbow limitations resulting from rheumatic diseases should be to achieve and maintain a pain-free functional arc of motion, which will improve function. This chapter reviews nonoperative management of arthritis of the elbow, preoperative evaluation, surgical treatment, and postoperative rehabilitation.

Nonsurgical Treatment

The mainstay of nonoperative management is optimum use of anti-inflammatory and antiremittive medications and occasional intra-articular injections of steroids. Use of steroid injections should be primarily aimed at patients with early stages of disease and active synovitis. Occupational and physical therapy for the patient with RA should include patient education; use of thermal modalities; maintenance of range of motion (ROM) and strength; ADL training; and instruction in the use of assistive devices, joint protection, and periodic splinting.

When elbow ROM is limited by acute or active synovitis, cold modalities are generally more effective than heat modalities for reducing inflammation. Cold packs made for this purpose or makeshift cold packs (such as a bag of frozen peas) placed on the elbow are one option. If this is too difficult for persons with polyarticular disease, J. L. Melvin (personal communication, December 8,

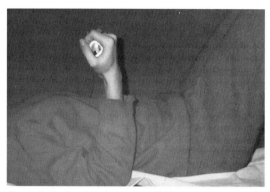 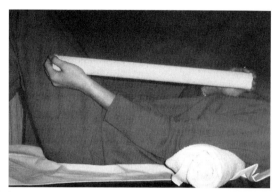

Figure 1. Supine dowel exercises. Patients are encouraged to maximize end-range elbow motion by stabilizing their shoulders against a bed, which helps to isolate the elbow and thus eliminates compensatory shoulder motion. The patient then uses the dowel for active assisted flexion (A) and extension (B).

1997) suggested having the patient dip the bent elbow in a container of refrigerated or iced water for 1 to 3 min. This is fast and can be more effective than poorly placed cold packs. Its efficiency allows patients to apply cold 4 to 6 times a day, which is more effective than the typical 1 to 2 applications of traditional cold packs.

When stiffness is the primary problem, heat is more effective. A heating pad is one option; performing ROM exercises in the shower under warm water is another. Thermal elbow sleeves or Heelbos™ (adaptAbility, Colchester, CT) can likewise warm the elbow and increase comfort.

Because elbow ROM is critical for upper-extremity function, active ROM exercises for flexion and extension, supination, and pronation should be performed once or twice daily for 10 slow repetitions to maintain or increase motion. The frequency and repetitions of these exercises depends on the patient's pain and endurance and the conditions of the joint.

In addition, gentle passive ROM may be initiated. Patients can use a dowel while lying supine and use the other arm to help the elbow extend and then flex. Working in one direction at a time (e.g., 10 repetitions in extension followed by 10 repetitions in flexion) appears to facilitate more range without increasing pain. This exercise can be performed against the wall by allowing the elbow to drop down by the side and using the dowel to bend the elbow into flexion. This position allows the patient to stabilize the shoulder to prevent substitution (Figure 1). Forearm rotation exercises with the dowel are achieved by keeping the elbow close to the side and having the patient use the other hand to assist the dowel (and therefore the forearm) into supination and then pronation. If any wrist limitations or hand deformities exist, these exercises may have to be adapted. For example, the wrist may need a wrist splint to provide support. The end of the dowel may be adapted to fit the hand deformity, or a strap may be added if grip is limited. One must caution the patient to work within his or her range of tolerance to avoid fatigue and increasing inflammation.

Isometric exercises for flexion, extension, supination, and pronation can be instituted once daily or every other day to maintain or improve muscle strength. The amount of repetition and length of muscle contraction will vary from patient to patient. A good starting point is 10 repetitions while holding for a count of 6 sec on each exercise. In general, heavy lifting is not appropriate. Isometric exercises without repetitive joint motion, together with functional use, are more than adequate strengthening for patients with arthritis.

Splints can be helpful in specific situations. The most common use of elbow splints is for treatment of ulnar neuropathy (Blackmore & Hotchkiss, 1995). In these cases, a volar elbow splint in 20° to 30° extension immobilizes the elbow to prevent motion from aggravating the nerve. The extended position deepens the cubital tunnel, thus reducing exposure of the nerve to pressure. Diamond and Lister (1985) and Blackmore and Hotchkiss (1995) recommend a volar long-arm splint that incorporates the wrist to relax the flexor carpi ulnaris muscle (see Blackmore & Hotchkiss, 1995 for a thorough review of this topic).

The rare patient with acute elbow synovitis that is unresponsive to rest, cold modalities, steroid injection, and anti-inflammatory medications may be more comfortable with a posterior custom thermoplastic splint, which is bubbled over the ulnar nerve and can be used when sleeping or at leisure. Use of a splint should be combined with cold modalities several times a day. Hinged splints have sometimes been used for symptomatic elbow instability; however, they are usually difficult to keep aligned with the axis of elbow rotation, and they limit forearm rotation (Driscoll, 1993). In addition, the weight of the brace may increase the demands placed on the shoulder, especially for the patient with rheumatoid arthritis.

Soft, padded elbow sleeves (Heelbo™) can play a substantial role in improving comfort for patients with inflammatory arthritis. Worn at night or during the day, elbow sleeves reduce pressure on the sensitive ulnar nerve, especially in persons with elbow flexion contractures. These sleeves can improve bed mobility by reducing pressure on painful nodules. Heelbos™ do not prevent motion or encourage elbow flexion contractures the way lamb's wool cuffs can, and they can be difficult to don for persons with fragile hands.

Preoperative Evaluation

Orthopedic Evaluation

Most patients with elbow arthritis are referred to surgery by a rheumatologist or internist and have received a full diagnostic workup. In most cases, the orthopedic examination confirms the referring diagnosis. If it does not, a diagnostic evaluation is initiated. At The Hospital for Special Surgery (New York, NY), a surgical scoring system for the elbow has been developed to facilitate evaluation and documentation of elbow function, pain, ROM, and strength both preoperatively and postoperatively (see Table 1) (Inglis & Pellicci, 1980).

Imaging and Additional Studies

The most useful imaging study of the elbow is standard radiography, which should consist of an anteroposterior view and a lateral view. Plain radiographs allow for accurate staging of rheumatic disease. By using the classification of Steinbrocker, Traeger, and Batterman (1949), Grade I disease consists of a mild to moderate synovitis with normal-appearing radiographs. Grade II disease involves persistent synovitis with radiographic evidence of mild joint-space narrowing. Grade III-A disease

Table 1. Preoperative Education Topics

The Hospital for Special Surgery: A Surgical Scoring System for the Elbow (30 points maximum)

Pain—30 points	Points	Flexifon contracture—6 points	Points
No pain at any time	30	Less than 15°	6
No pain when bending	15	Between 15 and 45°	4
Mild pain when bending	10	Between 45 and 90°	2
Moderate pain when bending	5	Greater than 90°	0
Severe pain when bending	0		
No pain at rest	15	**Extension contracture—6 points**	
Mild pain at rest	10	Greater than 120° flexion	6
Moderate pain at rest	5	100–120° flexion	4
Severe pain at rest	0	Less than 100°, greater than or equal to 80°	2
		Less than 80°	0
Function—20 points			
Bending activities for 30 min	8	**Pronation—4 points**	
Bending activities for 15 min	6	Greater than 60°	4
Bending activities for 5 min	4	Greater than 30–60°	3
Cannot use elbow	0	Greater than 15–30°	2
Unlimited use of elbow	12	Less than 0°	0
Limited only for recreation	10		
Household and employment	8	**Supination—4 points**	
Independent self-care	6	Greater than 60°	4
Invalid	0	Greater than 45–60°	3
		Greater than 15–45°	2
Saggital arc—20 points		Less than 15°	0
One point for each 7° arc of motion			
Muscle strength—10 points			
Can lift 5 lbs. (2.3 kg) to 90°	10		
Can lift 2 lbs. (0.9 kg) to 90°	8		
Arc of motion against gravity	5		
Cannot move through arc of motion	0		

Note. This surgical scoring system has been developed to facilitate evaluation and documentation of elbow function, pain, ROM, and strength (Inglis & Pellicci, 1980). From The Hospital for Special Surgery. New York, NY. Reprinted with permission.

involves a resolving synovitis but complete loss of joint space radiographically. Grade III-B disease involves loss of articular congruity with extensive subchrondral bone loss on radiographs and is usually associated with gross instability. Grade IV disease involves ankylosis of the joint.

Additional imaging studies such as magnetic resonance imaging (MRI), tomography, and computed tomography arthrography have a limited role in the evaluation of RA of the elbow. If there is a question regarding neurological involvement including ulnar neuropathy, an electromyography or nerve conduction study may be helpful.

Physical Therapy and Occupational Therapy Evaluation

In facilities where therapy evaluations are performed preoperatively, practitioners have the advantage of:

- evaluating preoperative function and the patient's compensatory or substitution patterns;
- educating the patient regarding the postoperative course so that she or he can plan for greater assistance with self-care, driving, and ADL (realistic preplanning greatly reduces postoperative stress for the patient); and
- training the patient in postoperative care, splint use, and exercises when he or she is not in postoperative pain or under the influence of anesthetics and analgesics.

Within the context of shortened length of stay, preoperative rehabilitation evaluation greatly facilitates a smooth postoperative course. A full evaluation should include the following information.

History. This includes age, hand dominance, medical and past surgical history, medications, social history, living arrangements, number of steps in the home, and ambulatory status. Both the onset of elbow involvement and of severe functional impairment are important to evaluate. The patient may have had elbow synovitis for 10 years but functional impairment for only 2 years. Medications including disease-modifying antirheumatic drugs and prednisone can often compromise skin quality and increase the risk of infection for this patient population (Figgie, Inglis, & Figgie, 1991).

Patient's plan for postoperative care. Who will assist the patient with basic self-care the first weeks after surgery? What sources or plan does he or she have for transportation, shopping, and so forth? What are the discharge plans?

Elbow ROM and strength. Both active and passive ROM must be evaluated. Elbow flexion or extension contractures should be noted because the patient with a severe elbow flexion contracture preoperatively may require immediate extension splinting to avoid recurrence or muscle reeducation to these contracted muscles. Patients often cannot elicit extensor muscle function after years of flexion contracture. Splinting can be initiated preoperatively to elongate muscles before surgery, providing the joint allows this. Even a 10° gain in extension is helpful. Supination and pronation are evaluated with the arm adducted to determine if the limitation is from the proximal radioulnar joint or the distal radioulnar joint. The source of the limitation is usually indicated by pain at the site of limitation after forearm rotation.

Elbow muscle function is evaluated with a manual muscle test. The ability to isolate elbow muscle function is likewise evaluated. Patients often use compensatory scapular and shoulder motion to elicit elbow extension or flexion. Initiation of exercises to isolate elbow flexion, extension, and forearm rotation before surgery facilitates postoperative rehabilitation.

Sensation. The ulnar nerve is vulnerable at the elbow for three reasons:

1. RA and OA frequently affect the cervical spine by creating pressure on the nerve roots, thereby altering nerve physiology and making the nerves more vulnerable to pressure distally (i.e., double crush syndrome; Osterman, 1988).

2. Synovitis and deformity at the ulnohumeral joint can entrap the ulnar nerve (Morrey, 1991).

3. Flexion contractures make the ulnar nerve more exposed to external pressure (Jones & Gauntt, 1979; McPherson & Meals, 1992).

Rarely, the radial nerve and the posterior interosseous nerve may be entrapped by synovitis (Morrey, 1991). Evaluation with the Semmes-Weinstein monofilaments is the most sensitive sensory test, but static and moving two-point discrimination can be used effectively to detect diminished sensation in the ulnar fingers secondary to nerve entrapment (Dellon, 1981; Weinstein, 1962). Evaluation of sensation to the dorsum of the little finger is the key area to test to distinguish between elbow (high) and wrist (low) compression of the ulnar nerve. The dorsal cutaneous branch is proximal to the wrist, and, therefore, if dorsal sensation to the little finger is diminished, the compression must be at the elbow. If the dorsum is intact and only volar sensation is diminished, the lesion must be at Guyon's canal or more distally (Dellon, 1981).

Evaluation of forces on the elbow. Limited shoulder, hip, or knee motion can refer large forces to the elbow joint during functional activities (Figgie et al., 1991). Limited shoulder motion transfers greater forces to the elbow. The use of ambulatory aids additionally increases stress across the elbow. It is critical to evaluate a patient's available ROM of proximal and distal joints so that a home program can be instituted to maximize this range, along with adaptive devices and ambulatory aides to minimize unnecessary forces to the elbow. This will be helpful if any future reconstructive arthroplasty is needed because these same forces have the potential of loosening or dislocating a TEA.

Function. At The Hospital for Special Surgery, each patient completes a questionnaire detailing functional limitations regarding ADL, level of pain, patient motivation, and level of desire to improve function. In addition, it is important to evaluate any compensatory substitution patterns the patient uses to accomplish a task (e.g., if the patient protracts the neck to accomplish feeding because of limited elbow flexion). This pattern may be aggravating coexistent cervical spine disease, or this substitution pattern may have increased the mobility of the neck. This substitution pattern must be controlled postoperatively to aim toward a goal of reaching the mouth via elbow flexion, not neck protraction.

Defining the exact functional needs of the patient is important in planning postoperative treatment and setting realistic postoperative goals. Likewise, ensuring that the surgeon, practitioner, and patient have the same goals and expectations before and after surgery is critical to obtain a successful outcome.

Surgery for RA

The surgical treatment options for the rheumatoid elbow include extra-articular soft-tissue procedures such as rheumatoid nodule or olecranon bursal excision and ulnar nerve transposition. Intra-articular procedures include synovectomy with or without radial head excision, fascial interposition arthroplasty, and TEA. The choice of treatment depends on the stage of disease and the functional needs of the patient. Preoperative evaluation by occupational and physical therapy practitioners can be extremely helpful for this patient population. Functional evaluation, patient education, and instruction in adaptive measures can greatly increase patient independence. Early involvement of the practitioner can additionally facilitate postoperative rehabilitation if later surgical intervention becomes necessary.

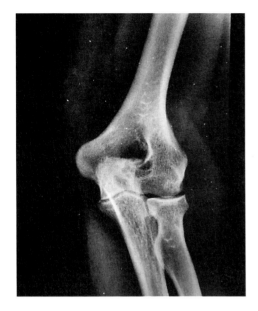

Figure 2. Stage II radiographic changes at the elbow. Radiograph of a patient with RA who is medically well controlled except for synovitis of the elbow. The patient is an excellent candidate for synovectomy.

Clinical Presentation

Patients with RA of the elbow most commonly present with pain and loss of motion at the elbow. Flexion and extension contractures are often present. Eventually, 20% to 50% of patients with RA will develop elbow involvement (see Figure 2, Porter, Park, Richardson, & Vainio, 1974). In the early stages of involvement, the clinical presentation is painful limitation of motion with associated swelling and synovitis. In later stages of disease, pain and limited motion result from joint destruction with loss of articular cartilage and subchondral bone. Further progression of bone and soft-tissue destruction can lead to instability. Patients with synovitis may present with symptoms related to ulnar neuropathy as the result of nerve compression in the cubital tunnel. In patients with JRA, ankylosis may be the end result.

Surgical Treatment of Periarticular Disease and Postoperative Rehabilitation

Stages of Wound Healing as a Guide to Postoperative Therapy

Rehabilitation of the rheumatoid elbow follows the principles of wound healing (Burkhalter, 1990; Madden, 1990). Understanding how the wound and body heal and form scars is essential to planning appropriate treatment for this or any patient population. The timeline for the different phases of healing is only a basic guideline. Healing is not always this precise, and planning should be individualized. A brief description of each phase of wound healing follows. For more detailed information, consult major hand therapy and surgery textbooks.

Inflammatory phase (1–7 days). This is both a vascular and cellular response to an injury (or, in this case, surgery) that produces the delivery of fluid to defend the body against alien substances.

Dead or dying tissue is disposed of, which prepares the tissue for the repair process. In this phase, for the first 5 days after surgery, the tensile strength of the wound is largely reliant on the epidermis and the sutures (Burkhalter, 1990; Smith, 1995). Logically, the focus of therapy during this phase is to rest, protect, elevate, and reduce edema. Gentle active, active-assisted, or passive ROM may be instituted, depending on the edema noted in the elbow and the status of the incision site. Ice is the main modality used. Retrograde massage is likewise helpful for reducing edema.

Fibroplasia phase (7–28 days). During this phase of wound healing, a restoration of mechanical integrity of the wound occurs through the migration of fibroblasts, which synthesize collagen and build the tensile strength of the wound (Burkhalter, 1990; Smith, 1995). From postoperative day (POD) 5 to POD 30, an increase in the tensile strength parallels the rise in collagen content in the wound. By 3 weeks after surgery, the normal incised and sutured wound has less than 15% of its ultimate tensile strength. It is not stronger because the collagen has not yet been organized. Therefore, during this phase of wound healing, it is important to maximize ROM and joint mobility and "model" the forming scar tissue while therapy can have some influence on its organization (Burkhalter, 1990; Smith, 1995). The focus of therapy is to maximize end ranges of elbow motion through prolonged gentle stretch, scar management, and increased functional use.

Scar maturation phase (28 days–1 year). During this phase, there is a prolonged period of metabolic activity in which the randomly oriented collagen fibers laid down in the fibroplasia phase become more organized and add strength to the wound (Burkhalter, 1990; Smith, 1995). The focus of therapy in this phase is to further maximize end ROM, to increase strength and endurance, and to maximize patient independence. Heat modalities may help reduce stiffness. In many cases, therapy after elbow surgery may not be necessary if early intervention is provided and the patient uses the arm in functional activities.

Olecranon Bursectomy

A chronically inflamed olecranon bursa that is unresponsive to conservative measures may require excision; this is referred to as an *olecranon bursectomy*. Although this may seem to be an innocuous procedure, the lack of subcutaneous tissue in this location increases the risk of wound-healing problems and infection. In addition, there may be a primary or secondary infection of the bursa. Therefore, routine cultures and pathology specimens should be examined at the time of excision. Patients undergoing rheumatoid nodule or olecranon bursal excision should be informed about the potential for wound-healing problems and the possibility of recurrence.

Rehabilitation: Olecranon Bursectomy

Hospitalization: Outpatient surgery. Inflammatory phase (1–7 days). Postoperatively, the elbow is generally splinted in a plaster half cast with a wrap for 7 to 14 days to allow wound healing. The elbow is elevated, and the patient is instructed to begin gentle ROM exercises to the shoulder, wrist, and hand. Adaptive devices may be issued to increase independence in self-care during elbow immobilization. The most common complication of olecranon bursectomy is wound dehiscence (i.e., having the wound split open) (Kerr, 1993). Thus, therapy for elbow ROM is usually postponed until wound healing occurs and the surgeon inspects the wound and removes the stitches on approximately POD 10 to 14.

Fibroplasia phase (7–28 days). Once the wound has healed, retrograde massage as needed and gentle scar massage can be initiated. Special care not to aggravate the skin of the scar is needed to prevent or reduce the risk of infection. Compressive garments may be used to control soft-tissue swelling. Ice is used with caution to avoid pressure or to avoid compromising skin quality at the wound. Active ROM consisting of elbow flexion, extension, pronation, and supination is generally started after immobilization is carried over into general functional use of the elbow. Careful observation of the wound is essential. The patient is instructed to avoid pressure on the elbow olecranon area. Local protective padding for the elbow, especially with tasks that require leaning or pressure on the elbow, is encouraged (Kerr, 1993). Exercises should be discontinued and a physician consulted if the wound becomes swollen, erythematous, or spontaneously drains. The amount and duration of therapy will depend on limitations that occur in this phase. Generally, a strong home program of 3 to 4 daily ROM exercises of 10 repetitions each combined with functional use is sufficient. Outpatient therapy is indicated when there are major limitations.

Scar maturation phase (28 days–1 year). Therapy is not usually necessary in this phase unless contractures develop. Possible serial static splinting to maximize end ROM may be indicated.

Ulnar Nerve Transposition

Occasionally, patients with inflammatory arthritis of the elbow present with ulnar neuropathy. The ulnar neuropathy is often secondary to extension of the synovitis and results in compression of the ulnar nerve in the cubital tunnel. The surgical treatment involves anterior transposition of the ulnar nerve in combination with a synovectomy and radial head excision through a posterior triceps-sparing approach.

Rehabilitation: Ulnar Nerve Transposition

Hospitalization: Day of surgery or inpatient 2 to 5 days. Inflammatory phase (1–7 days). Postoperatively, the elbow is immobilized in a plaster splint in 30° of flexion for the first 24 to 48 hr. After a brief immobilization period, active ROM is initiated and upgraded according to the patient's tolerance. Cold modalities (5–7 min) are usually used 3 to 4 times a day. Splinting is generally not necessary, and a sling may be used for comfort. Elbow flexion, extension, supination, and pronation exercises are issued (in writing) for home use 3 to 4 times daily with 10 to 20 repetitions as necessary. Functional use is encouraged with a weight limit of 3 to 5 lbs. for the first 6 to 8 weeks to protect the triceps repair.

If a submuscular transposition of the ulnar nerve is performed, a longer period of immobilization is required. A long-arm splint with the wrist included to protect the origins of the flexor and pronator muscles is necessary. Because of the longer immobilization required, this type of transposition is generally not performed for the patient with RA (Figgie, Inglis, Mow, & Figgie, 1989a).

Fibroplasia and scar maturation phase. Prolonged outpatient therapy is seldom necessary if early mobilization is initiated and the patient follows through with a complete home program. For some patients, hypersensitivity of the scar may need desensitization. Nerve gliding can be instituted in the inflammatory phase and continued at this stage.

Surgical Treatment of Intra-Articular Disease and Postoperative Rehabilitation

Synovectomy

Synovectomy, or removal of synovial pannus from the elbow joint, is effective for uncontrolled synovitis where there is preservation of the articular cartilage (Figure 3). The primary indications for synovectomy include painful synovitis in an elbow in the early stages of disease (Stage I or II) for which 6 months of optimal medical management has failed to control the synovitis. Although synovectomy can be performed in later stages of disease (Stage III-A), the results are less predictable (Inglis, Ranawat, & Straub, 1971). Patients with severe joint destruction (Stage III-B) or marked limitation of motion are not candidates for synovectomy.

Synovectomy is particularly beneficial for patients in whom the inflammatory disease is well controlled medically with the exception of one or two joints. Synovectomy of the recalcitrant joint or joints may allow the patient to maintain medical control of the disease after synovectomy with lower levels of disease-modifying drugs.

The primary goal of synovectomy is to provide pain relief with improvement in function as a secondary goal. Patients must be informed that improvement in ROM after synovectomy is unpredictable and, although important to function, is not the primary goal. If ROM is greatly limited, then other surgical options such as TEA should be considered.

Synovectomy of the elbow, although effective, is a palliative procedure. Patients should understand that the synovium regenerates after synovectomy. Therefore, recurrent synovitis requiring repeat synovectomy and further joint destruction requiring TEA are distinct possibilities.

Although it is a controversial procedure, most of the time radial head excision is performed as part of the synovectomy. Excision of the radial head allows for improved exposure for performing the synovectomy and allows for relief of painful, proximal forearm rotation. This is generally accomplished through a lateral (Kocher) incision. However, as mentioned previously, if the patient has concomitant symptoms of ulnar nerve compression, a posterior triceps-sparing approach is used that allows the surgeon to perform an ulnar nerve transposition, radial head excision, and synovectomy with a single approach.

Pain relief after synovectomy is predictable, with 75% to 80% of patients reporting satisfactory pain relief (Inglis et al., 1971). However, ROM after synovectomy is less predictable. For approximately 40% of patients, ROM will improve; for another 40%, it will not change; and for 20%, it will decrease. Decreased ROM is more likely in patients with JRA or patients with limited preoperative ROM. Postsynovectomy follow-up at 10 to 20 years has shown slow deterioration of results regarding pain relief and ROM (Alexiades, Stanwyck, Figgie, & Inglis, 1990). However, despite the deterioration of results, relatively few patients required further surgery (Alexiades et al., 1990). One of the factors affecting long-term results is the tendency for patients to develop instability of the elbow over time because of progressive joint disease (Alexiades et al., 1990) (Figure 4). This results in functional loss of strength at the elbow and difficulty performing overhead activities.

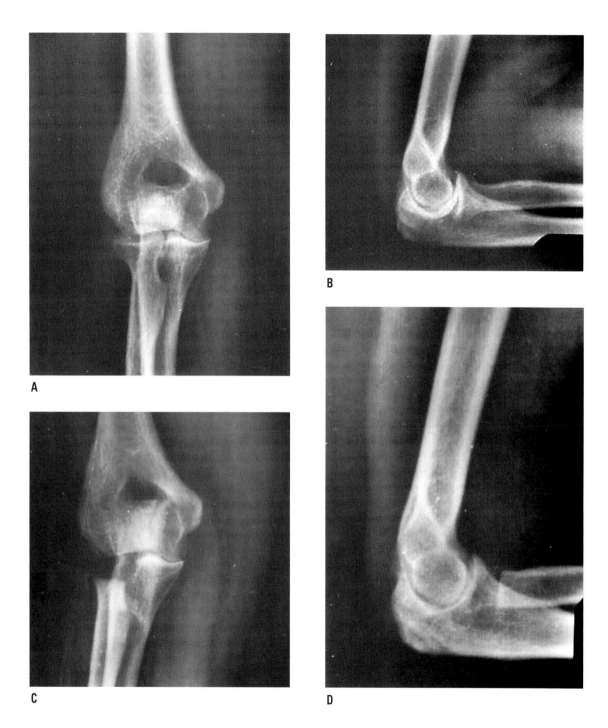

Figure 3. Synovectomy for RA. The patient had Stage III-A radiographic changes of her elbow and marked disability (A, B). She was successfully treated with a radial head excision and elbow synovectomy (C, D).

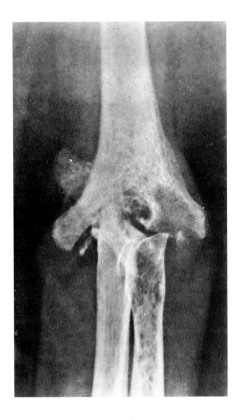

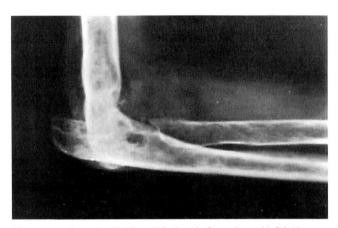

Figure 4. Radiographs (A left, and B above) of a patient with RA 15 years after treatment with synovectomy. Despite the marked joint destruction that has occurred, this patient had no pain and was satisfied with the results.

Complications after synovectomy are rare. Wound-healing problems may develop, but the risk of infection is low. Postoperative fracture may occur, but it too is rare. Ulnar nerve injury is possible but uncommon. Loss of motion may occur postoperatively; this usually results from poor patient selection or failure to adhere to postoperative rehabilitation.

Rehabilitation: Synovectomy

Hospitalization: Day of surgery or inpatient 1–5 days. Inflammatory phase (1–7 days). Rehabilitation after synovectomy is of vital importance. Patients often spend 3 to 5 days in the hospital after an open synovectomy to undergo intensive therapy. Patients (without infection or wound closure problems) may begin with a continuous passive motion (CPM) machine immediately after their surgery (Figure 5). The surgery is performed with a regional anesthetic to avoid the risk of general anesthesia and to allow the patient to begin ROM exercises while the arm is still anesthetized. Ice, elevation, and retrograde massage are used to minimize edema. The patient is examined on the first or second postoperative day to begin gentle active and active assisted ROM exercises, typically 3

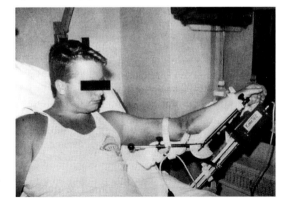

Figure 5. A CPM machine can be used postoperatively to assist patients in increasing ROM.

times a day with 10 repetitions of each exercise. The patient is issued a sling for rest and is encouraged to use the arm for ADL. Staples are removed on POD 10 to 12, depending on wound closure.

Fibroplasia phase (7–28 days). If a major contracture was noted preoperatively, it is often necessary to use gentle static progressive splinting such as an elbow extension brace or a flexion brace. We use a design created at The Hospital for Special Surgery (Figure 6). These braces are usually fabricated in occupational therapy once the wound has healed and swelling has decreased on or about POD 10. The braces produce a low force that results in slow progressive stretching, in turn producing tissue elongation (sometimes referred to as plastic deformation) at low peak loads (Bonutti, Windau, Ables, & Miller, 1994). Dynamic splinting is too forceful and often results in increased inflammation, discomfort, and decreased ROM. The static progressive splint is worn at night or when the patient is resting so that functional use of the elbow is maximized during the day. For patients with polyarticular disease, the splint may be adapted with straps to facilitate donning and doffing, or caregivers may need instruction to help the patient. If the patient is having difficulty with cocontracture and eliciting the biceps or triceps to contract, biofeedback can be extremely helpful in regaining this function. Facilitation or massage to the biceps and or triceps while the patient attempts to achieve end ROM can likewise encourage relaxation and maximal range.

Scar maturation phase (28 days–1 year). Splinting to increase functional ROM is continued at night until improvement plateaus and a hard end feel is noted. Strengthening is achieved through active use rather than specific exercises.

Total Elbow Arthroplasty

Improvements in implant design, surgical technique, and understanding of the importance of alignment have all contributed to more predictable outcomes with TEA (Figgie, Inglis, & Mow, 1986). Early total elbow designs consisted of constrained hinges that developed rapid loosening and resulted in implant failure. In addition, high complication rates were reported with the constrained designs, including infection, wound-healing problems, and ulnar neuropathy. Improvements in surgical technique have greatly reduced the rate of complications.

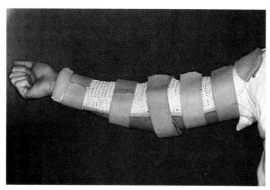 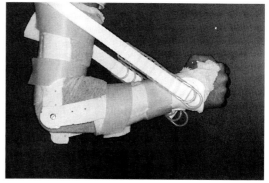

Figure 6. In the fibroplasia phase of wound healing, an extension brace (A) or a flexion brace (B) facilitates maximum end ROM. Patients are instructed to wear braces at night or 2 to 3 times a day for 1 to 2 hours at a time.

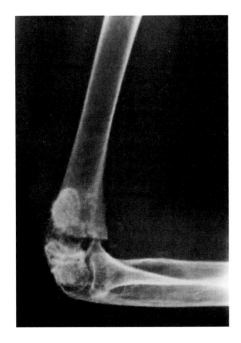
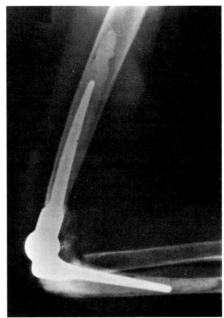

Figure 7. This patient had a supracondylar nonunion that left her with a flail elbow (A, left). She underwent a TEA with an excellent clinical result (B, right).

Surgical Indications

The primary indications for TEA include pain, limited ROM, and advanced stages of arthritis radiographically (Stages III-A, III-B, and IV). Patients with inflammatory arthritis are ideal candidates for TEA. Contraindications to TEA include active infection, neuropathic joint disease, or a flail elbow secondary to neurological injury or neuromuscular disease. Hemophilia is a relative contraindication because of an increased risk of major bleeding, wound-healing problems, and infection.

Patients with ankylosis (Stage IV) of the elbow experience great functional loss and limitation in ADL, including the inability to reach their face and loss of independence in personal hygiene. Therefore, TEA is performed in selected patients with ankylosis in an attempt to improve ROM and function. Despite the duration of ankylosis, an average of 80° of flexion and extension can be achieved, which results in great functional improvement that allows patients to care for themselves (Figgie, Inglis, Mow, & Figgie, 1989a).

Another infrequent indication for TEA is supracondylar fracture or fracture nonunion, particularly involving an elbow with inflammatory arthritis. Fracture fixation may be limited by the quality of bone, and further functional disability may result from periarticular fibrosis. TEA therefore may be the most appropriate treatment allowing for immediate functional use of the elbow. These are technically difficult procedures and should be considered a "salvage operation" (Figure 7).

Implant Design Considerations

Contemporary designs of TEA include nonconstrained and semiconstrained devices. The nonconstrained devices, such as the capitello-condylar implant, rely on the integrity of soft tissues for stability. Therefore, use of this type of implant requires that the patient have intact ligamentous support and sufficient bone stock (Figure 8). Nonconstrained implants are more difficult to insert and may have less application because there will often be major bone loss or ligamentous instability by the time TEA is indicated in most patients. The theoretical advantage of unconstrained devices is that there is less stress on the bone cement interface that may result in less frequent loosening. However, with this type of prosthesis, instability is often a greater problem because of the difficulties with soft-tissue balancing and problems with polyethylene wear. In addition, ulnar nerve problems may be more frequent because the nerve is often not exposed with the lateral approach.

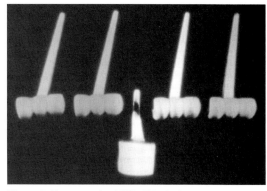

Figure 8. Nonconstrained TEA. This device relies on adequate bone stock and soft-tissue support for stability.

Semiconstrained implants usually have a locking-hinge mechanism that prevents subluxation or dislocation. Although semiconstrained devices theoretically may have increased rates of loosening from increased stress transfer to the bone cement interface, this has not been observed in our clinical experience (Figgie, Inglis, Mow, Ranawat, & Figgie, 1990). The main advantage of semiconstrained implants is their more universal application. The intrinsic stability in semiconstrained devices broadens the application to include patients with poor ligamentous support and severe bone loss. In addition, semiconstrained devices are technically more forgiving and allow for more predictable results with a lower complication rate (Figure 9).

Improvements in function and ROM have been achieved largely through improved implant design and understanding the importance of restoring the center of rotation of the elbow. The ability to restore the center of rotation allows for more normal elbow kinematics and improved function of the muscles at the elbow, which results in improved ROM. Occasionally, custom

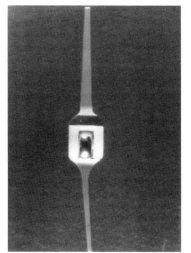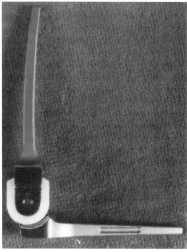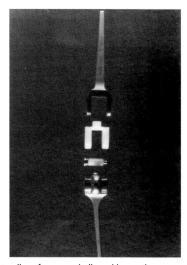

Figure 9. A semiconstrained TEA such as the ones pictured (A, B, C) has built-in laxity to allow for normal elbow kinematics. However, because of the intrinsic stability of the device, its use is not dependent on soft-tissue integrity and is less dependent on bone stock. The current design helps restore anatomical alignment (B). The disassembled view (C) shows the non–load-bearing restraining axle that provides the device with intrinsic stability.

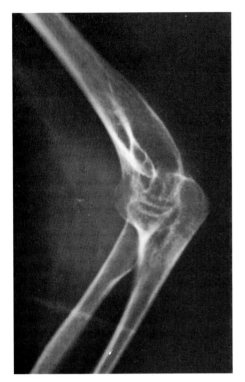

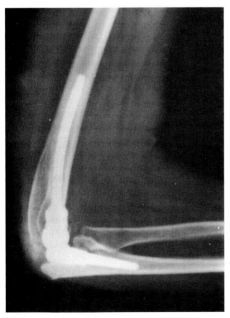

Figure 10. Adolescent patient with JRA ankylosis of both elbows (A above). She was dependent for all ADL. The patient was successfully treated with bilateral custom TEAs (B below). The patient gained a 100° arc of motion in each elbow and was independent in ADL.

implants may be required to restore the anatomy of the elbow. The need for custom implants is most common in patients with JRA who have small bone size and occasionally marked bone deformity resulting from premature closure of the growth plates (Figure 10).

Outcomes and Complications

The results of 137 TEAs performed in patients with RA revealed a satisfactory outcome in 125 patients and good to excellent results in 105 patients (Figgie, Inglis, Mow, Ranawat, & Figgie, 1990. The average follow-up was greater than 6 years, with the longest being 13 years. The average postoperative range of motion was 103° of flexion and extension and 130° of forearm rotation (Figure 10). The reported postoperative complications included deep infection in 4 elbows, postoperative epicondylar fractures in 7 elbows, and wound problems in 7 elbows. There were 12 failures—4 for deep infection and 8 for late dislocation. The 8 with late dislocation underwent satisfactory revisions. The problem of dislocation resulted from a snap-fit type of design. The design was subsequently modified from a snap-fit to an axle type, which eliminated the possibility of dislocation. Five-year survivorship in 86 TEAs with the recent design change was 90% for patients with RA (Kraay, Figgie, Wolfe, & Ranawat, 1994).

The rates of complication for TEA have decreased. Improvements in surgical technique, including use of a posteromedial surgical approach, have resulted in fewer complications related to wound healing. In addition, the use of the posteromedial approach (Bryan & Morrey, 1982) has virtually eliminated any problems with the triceps mechanism and the ulnar nerve in patients with inflammatory arthropathy. The posteromedial triceps-sparing approach allows for early initiation of therapy, thus improving ROM and functional outcome. Despite improved motion, patients rarely obtain full extension and are forewarned to expect a 15 to 30° flexion contracture. Careful placement of incisions to avoid pressure points, particularly in patients requiring assistive devices for ambulation, reduces the risk of wound-healing problems. The risk of infection, historically 6 to 13%, has decreased dramatically with the change in surgical approach and the routine use of antibiotic-impregnated cement. In addition, patients with American College of Rheumatology Class IV adult rheumatoid arthritis disease and patients with psychiatric problems are at higher risk for infection (Wolfe, Figgie, Inglis, Bonn, & Ranawat, 1990).

Postoperative epicondylar fractures may occur, but careful surgical technique and modifications in implant design have reduced the risk of fracture. If an epicondylar fracture occurs, healing usually ensues with treatment in a brace that does not compromise the final result.

Rehabilitation: Semiconstrained TEA

Hospitalization: Inpatient 2 to 5 days. Postoperative management varies widely. One author (M.P.F.) keeps the patient in the hospital to start CPM, fabricate splints, and begin therapy on POD 2. Other surgeons discharge the patient on POD 2 in a plaster half cast with the elbow in 70 to 80° flexion and have the elbow examined in outpatient therapy on POD 3 or 4.

The following is a list of precautions and considerations in rehabilitation.

- Rupture of the triceps: avoid resistive extension for the first 4 weeks after surgery.
- Infection or delayed healing: carefully observe the incision for drainage and red or warm areas.
- Ulnar nerve compression: evaluate sensation and observe motor loss in the ulnar nerve distribution.
- Patient is not to lift more than 1 lb. during the first 3 months after surgery.

Inflammatory phase (1–7 days). Postoperatively, the patient is initially placed in a well-padded, posterior, plaster elbow splint at approximately 30° of extension for the first 2 days. ROM for the shoulder and hand is initiated. Once adequate wound healing is achieved, the patient begins active assisted, active, and gentle passive ROM, including flexion–extension and pronation–supination exercises. A hinged, static, progressive splint (Hospital for Special Surgery design) is fabricated by occupational therapy and fitted on approximately POD 2 if wound is healing without complication (Figure 11). The splint is used to protect the incision and to assist in obtaining maximum flexion and extension. The wrist may or may not be included for comfort if function is not compromised by restricting wrist motion. Velcro® straps applied to the brace allow for strapping the elbow in either end-range flexion or extension while at rest, depending on which motion is limited. If ulnar nerve symptoms are present, this splint can be left in extension (–15° to –30°) to alleviate pressure at the cubital tunnel area. During the first 1 to 2 weeks, soft-tissue swelling is managed with cold

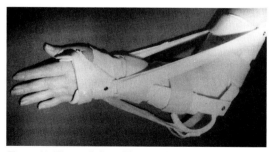 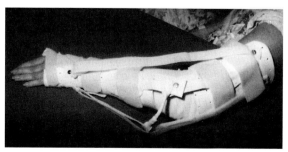

Figure 11. The total elbow hinge static progressive splint provides support to the elbow after surgery and protects the incision site. In addition, the splint can be positioned in either flexion (A) or extension (B), depending on the needs of the patient.

modalities, elevation, retrograde massage, and compressive wraps or garments. The practitioner should pay careful attention to the wound during this early phase of healing. Any drainage or change in wound appearance should be noted and the surgeon notified. In some cases, exercise may need to be discontinued and the elbow splinted in extension until healing occurs. The triceps-sparing approach allows for early active and gentle passive ROM beginning on POD 2 or 3. The patient is instructed to perform active and active assisted ROM exercises 3 to 4 times per day to the elbow and 2 times a day to the shoulder and wrist. Gentle passive ROM exercises performed by the practitioner may be initiated once daily, along with CPM to maximize end ROM. Passive motion should be executed with great care. Aggressive passive motion exercises can lead to increased inflammation and, in the flexed position, triceps rupture or avulsion. A slow gentle stretch, massage, and concentrating on one motion at a time is most effective with this patient population. Resistive extension (e.g., pushing up from a chair, use of crutches) is prohibited to protect the triceps attachment.

When not exercising or using the elbow in the splint for functional activities, a CPM device is used to maximize available motion of the elbow. The splint is positioned at night in either flexion or extension to maximize motion that may be lacking. The patient is instructed to use the CPM machine independently and to increase the range gradually. Any increase in swelling, pain, or onset of paraesthesias should be monitored closely by the nursing staff members and patient. The amount of time spent in the CPM machine varies depending on the active and passive ROM, the status of the incision, and the amount of functional use. Initially, the CPM machine is set up for night use and for as many hours during the day as ROM and functional exercises will allow. If adequate ROM (40–100°) is achieved in the first few days, the patient may use the CPM machine only at night. There are no studies that validate the effectiveness of CPM for increasing ROM in a TEA. If no CPM machine is available, the patient may increase active ROM in his or her home program as necessary to improve limited motion.

Precautions, including avoidance of resistive extension, are reviewed with the patient before discharge. Basic hygiene and feeding activities are encouraged while in the hospital. ROM at the end of the hospital stay should range from 40° to 100° flexion with 70° of pronation and supination. The patient is discharged with the CPM for night use, the splint, and a full home program of active and passive ROM exercises.

Fibroplasia phase (7–28 days). Outpatient therapy starts anywhere from the 5th to the 10th day, depending on the surgeon. The splint continues to be worn for protection and is used to regain maximal end ranges. Other serial static splint options may include a static dorsal extension splint, a static progressive flexion, or an extension splint as previously discussed. Always keep in mind that degrees of motion are not the primary goal for this patient population, and splinting is used when functional use is compromised. Active and passive ROM is gained through moist heat and stretch. Heating the patient in one direction, flexion, or extension then working in the same direction is most productive. Massage to the bicep and tricep muscles helps to relax and reduce possible muscle spasms. Many of these patients have had flexion or extension contractures and experience extrinsic muscle shortening, which must be addressed in therapy.

Scar maturation phase (28 days–1 year). Splinting and ROM exercises are generally continued for 4 to 6 weeks at home postoperatively and then discontinued unless function remains limited. Strengthening or weight training is not appropriate for this patient population. Active use and gentle

Theraband™ (Hygenic Corp., Akron, OH) or isometric exercises are adequate for maximizing strength. Patients are generally advised to avoid lifting anything more than 1 lb. during the first 3 months and no more than 5 lb thereafter.

Rehabilitation: Nonconstrained TEA

Hospitalization: Inpatient 2 to 5 days. The following are precautions and consideration in rehabilitating nonconstrained TEA (Ewald et al., 1993).

- Dislocation or instability: lateral torque of any kind should be avoided. No combined shoulder abduction with elbow extension is allowed for 4 to 6 weeks postoperatively.
- Infection or delayed wound healing: observe incision area closely for drainage, redness, or warmth and report to the surgeon.
- Ulnar nerve compression: evaluate ulnar nerve distribution.

Inflammatory phase (1–7 days). The rehabilitation for nonconstrained devices differs from constrained devices in that the periods of immobilization tend to be longer (up to 3–4 weeks) and the initiation of ROM is more controlled and gradual. Consequently, nonconstrained devices need little rehabilitation. Recommended immobilization is with a prefabricated orthosis in 30 to 40° of flexion. A sling is used to hold the arm in adduction. After a few days, active ROM is initiated for flexion and extension. Supination and pronation may or may not be instituted if stability is questionable; this should be determined by the surgeon. Particular care must be taken in introducing supination because it places stress on the lateral ligament repair. If the elbow continues to be stable, the splint is discontinued within the first week. Weiland and associates (Davis, Weiland, Hungerford, Moore, & Volenec-Dowling, 1982; Weiland, Weiss, Wills, & Moore, 1989) recommend a posterior splint in 90° of flexion and in neutral forearm rotation. For the first 3 to 5 days, only passive ROM is recommended. Linscheid (1991) recommended casting for 3 to 4 weeks and subsequent splinting for a total of 6 weeks. The patient can use the hand as long as it is adducted and she or he does not lift anything more than 1 to 2 lb.

Fibroplasia and scar maturation phase. Depending on the period of immobilization, therapy may be necessary to increase ROM. At Brigham and Women's Hospital (Boston, MA), early controlled active ROM is recommended with minimal therapy intervention. If a longer period of immobilization is required for maintaining the stability of the elbow joint, static progressive splinting may be necessary. Elbow-extension splinting should be used with caution because it can cause dislocation of an unstable elbow. In general, motion is gained through functional use of the elbow. Patient education to avoid shoulder abduction combined with elbow extension for 6 months is stressed throughout pre- and postoperative care (Ewald et al., 1993).

Alternative Procedures: Arthrodesis, Distraction, and Resection Arthroplasties

Arthrodesis, or fusion, of the elbow results in major functional disability for the patient. Unfortunately, there is not an ideal position in which to arthrodese the elbow. The loss of motion that results from an arthrodesis decreases the ability to perform ADL. Particularly disabling is the inability of patients to move their hand to their face. In addition, a solid arthrodesis can be difficult to obtain in patients with inflammatory arthritis. Furthermore, a solid arthrodesis results in a transfer of greater stresses to the adjacent joints and, if achievable, places greater stress on the ipsilateral joints.

Therefore, elbow arthrodesis has limited indications, namely for a young patient who requires a pain-free elbow for manual labor. Even patients with infection may be better served with a resection arthroplasty, which will often function like a synovectomy and provide adequate pain relief and stability (Figgie, Inglis, Mow, Wolfe, Sculco, & Figgie, 1990).

Distraction arthroplasty is a procedure primarily designed to increase ROM in a stiff elbow. This is accomplished by performing an extensive soft-tissue release, often both intra-articular and extra-articular, followed by placement of a special hinged external fixator. The hinged external fixators provide immediate stability and allow for immediate ROM. By distracting the joint, they help to gain motion and prevent intra-articular adhesions. When the articular cartilage has been greatly damaged, a fascial interposition is performed in addition to the distraction arthroplasty. The fascia is attached to the articular joint surface to provide a membrane that effectively replaces the cartilage. Distraction arthroplasty with or without fascial interposition is primarily indicated in the patient with posttraumatic arthritis of the elbow. The rehabilitation process is extensive and similar to the postoperative rehabilitation for elbow synovectomy.

Resection arthroplasty, as the term implies, involves resecting or removing the joint. This operation has little or no role as a primary method of treatment for RA of the elbow. However, it does provide for reasonable salvage of an infected TEA. As mentioned previously, it can provide reasonable pain relief; however, function is usually limited by instability (Figgie, Inglis, Mow, Wolfe, Sculco, & Figgie, 1990).

Summary

There are many treatment options to offer the patient with severe elbow involvement as a result of RA. Deciding which treatments are best for these patients depends on the stage of the disease and functional limitations of the patient as well as the patient's functional demands, expectations, and compliance. Successful outcome of both nonsurgical and surgical treatment is dependent on good communication among the surgeon, the patient, and the rehabilitation team to set realistic goals and expectations.

References

Alexiades, M. M., Stanwyck, T. S., Figgie, M. P., & Inglis, E. (1990). Minimum ten year follow-up of elbow synovectomy for rheumatoid arthritis. *Orthopedic Transcripts, 14*, 255.

Blackmore, S. M., & Hotchkiss, R. N. (1995). Therapist's management of ulnar neuropathy at the elbow. In L. H. Hunter, E. J. Mackin, & A. D. Callahan (Eds.), *Rehabilitation of the hand* (4th ed.). St. Louis, MO: Mosby.

Bonutti, P. M., Windau, J. E., Ables, B. A., & Miller, B. G. (1994). Static progressive stretch to re-establish elbow ROM. *Clinical Orthopaedics and Related Research, 303*, 128–134.

Bryan, R. S., & Morrey, B. F. (1982). Extensive posterior exposure of the elbow: A triceps-sparing approach. *Clinical Orthopaedics and Related Research, 166*, 188–192.

Burkhalter, W. E. (1990). Wound classification and management. In J. M. Hunter, L. H. Schneider, E. J. Mackin, & A. D. Callahan (Eds.), *Rehabilitation of the hand* (3rd ed.). St. Louis, MO: Mosby.

Davis, R. F., Weiland, A. J., Hungerford, D. S., Moore, R. J., & Volenec-Dowling, S. (1982). Nonconstrained total elbow arthroplasty. *Clinical Orthopedics and Related Research, 171,* 156–160.

Dellon, A. L. (1981). *Evaluation of sensibility and re-education of the sensation in the hand.* Baltimore: Williams & Wilkins.

Diamond, M. L. & Lister, G. D. (1985). Cubital tunnel syndrome treated by long-arm splintage [abstract]. *Journal of Hand Surgery, 10A,* 430.

Driscoll, S. W. (1993). Surgery of elbow arthritis. In D. J. MacCarthy & W. J. Koopman (Eds.), *Arthritis and allied conditions: A textbook of rheumatology* (12th ed.). Baltimore: Williams & Wilkins.

Ewald, F. C., Simmons, E. D., Sullivan, J. R., Thomas, W. H., Scott, R. D., Poss, R., Thornhill, T. S., & Sledge, C. B. (1993). Capitellocondylar total elbow replacement in rheumatoid arthritis: Long term results. *Journal of Bone and Joint Surgery, 75A,* 498–507.

Figgie, M. P., Inglis, A. E., & Figgie, H. E. (1991). Total elbow athroplasty. In W. Petty (Ed.), *Total joint replacement* (pp. 659–706). Philadelphia: Saunders.

Figgie, H. E. III, Inglis, A. E., & Mow, C. S. (1986). A critical analysis of biomechanical factors affecting functional outcome in total elbow arthoplasties. *Journal of Arthroplasty, 1,* 169–73.

Figgie, M. P., Inglis, A. E., Mow, C. S., & Figgie, H. E. III. (1989a). Total elbow arthroplasty for complete ankylosis of the elbow. *Journal of Bone and Joint Surgery, 71A,* 513–520.

Figgie, M. P., Inglis, A. E., Mow, C. S., & Figgie, H. E. III. (1989b). Salvage of nonunion of supracondalar fracture of the humerus by elbow. *Journal of Bone and Joint Surgery, 71A,* 1058–1065.

Figgie, M. P., Inglis, A. E., Mow, C. S., Ranawat, C. S., & Figgie, H. E. III. (1990). Semi-constrained total elbow arthroplasty in rheumatoid arthritis. *Orthopedic Transcripts, 14,* 104.

Figgie, M. P., Inglis, A. E., Mow, C. S., Wolfe, S. W., Sculco, T. P., & Figgie, H. E. III. (1990). Results of reconstruction for failed total elbow arthroplasty. *Clinical Orthopaedics and Related Research, 253,* 123.

Goodfellow, J. W., & Bullough, P. B. (1967). The pattern of aging of the articular cartilage of the elbow joint. *Journal of Bone and Joint Surgery, 49B,* 175–181.

Inglis, A. E., & Pellicci, P. M. (1980). Total elbow replacement. *Journal of Bone and Joint Surgery, 62A,* 1252–1258.

Inglis, A. E., Ranawat, C. S., & Straub, L. B. (1971). Synovectomy and debridement of the elbow in rheumatoid arthritis. *Journal of Bone and Joint Surgery, 53A,* 652–662.

Jones, R. E., & Gauntt, C. (1979). Medial epicondylectomy for the ulnar nerve compression syndrome at the elbow. *Clinical Orthopaedics and Related Research, 139,* 174–178.

Kerr, D. R. (1993, January). Prepatellar and olecranon arthroscopic bursectomy. *Clinics in Sports Medicine, 12*(1), 137–142.

Linscheid, R. (1991). Unconstrained devices, techniques and results. In B. E. Morrey (Ed.), *Joint replacement arthroplasty* (pp. 293–309). New York: Churchill Livingstone.

Madden, J. W. (1990). Wound healing: The biological basis of hand surgery. In J. M. Hunter, S. L. H. Schneider, E. J. Mackin, & A. D. Callahan (Eds.), *Rehabilitation of the hand* (3rd ed.). St. Louis, MO: Mosby.

McPherson, S. A., & Meals, R. A. (1992). Cubital tunnel syndrome. *Orthopedic Clinics of North America 23*(1), 111–123.

Morrey, B. E. (Ed.). (1991). Joint replacement arthroplasty. In B. E. Morrey (Ed.), *Joint replacement arthroplasty* (pp. 243–382). New York: Churchill Livingstone.

Morrey, B. E., Askew, L. J., An, K. N., & Chao, E. Y. (1981). A biomechanical study of normal functional elbow motion. *Journal of Bone and Joint Surgery, 63A*, 87–89.

Osterman, A. L. (1988). The double crush syndrome. *Orthopedic Clinics of North America, 19*(1), 147–155.

Porter, B. B., Park, N., Richardson, C., & Vainio, K. (1974). Rheumatoid arthritis of the elbow: The results of synovectomy. *Journal of Bone and Joint Surgery, 56B*, 427–437.

Smith, K. (1995). Wound care for the hand patient. In L. H. Hunter, E. J. Mackin, & A. D. Callahan (Eds.), *Rehabilitation of the hand* (4th ed., pp. 237–250). St. Louis, MO: Mosby.

Steinbrocker, O., Traeger, C. H., & Batterman, R. C. (1949). Therapeutic criteria in rheumatoid arthritis. *Journal of the American Medical Association, 140*, 659–665.

Weiland, A. J., Weiss, A. P., Wills, R. P., & Moore, J. R. (1989). Capitello-condylar total elbow replacement: A long term follow-up study. *Journal of Bone and Joint Surgery, 71A*, 217–222.

Weinstein, S. (1962). Tactile sensitivity in the phalanges. *Perceptual Motor Skills, 14*, 351–354.

Wolfe, S. W., Figgie, M. P., Inglis, A. E., Bonn, W. W., & Ranawat, C. S. (1990). Management of infection about total elbow prosthesis. *Journal of Bone and Joint Surgery, 72A*, 198–212.

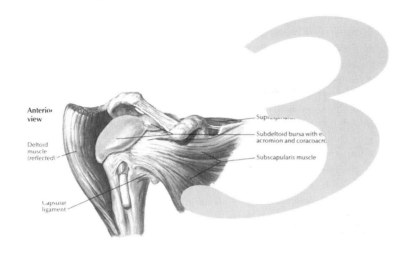

Anterior
view

Deltoid
muscle
(reflected)

Capsular
ligament

Supraspinatus

Subdeltoid bursa with e.
acromion and coracoacro

Subscapularis muscle

SHOULDER SURGERY AND REHABILITATION

*Thomas S. Thornhill, MD, Victoria Gall, MEd, PT, Susan Vermette, OTR,
and Frances Griffin, RN, BSN*

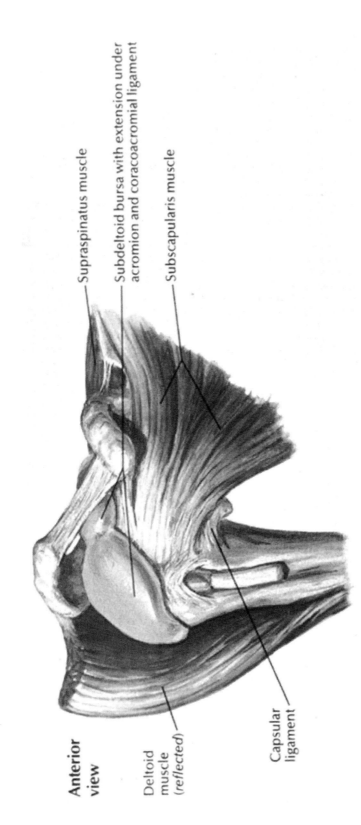

Anterior
view

Supraspinatus muscle

Subdeltoid bursa with extension under
acromion and coracoacromial ligament

Subscapularis muscle

Deltoid
muscle
(reflected)

Capsular
ligament

Anatomy of the shoulder—anterior view. Copyright 1989. Novartis. Reprinted with permission from the *Atlas of Human Anatomy*, illustrated by Frank H. Netter, MD. All rights reserved.

The pioneering work of Dr. Charles Neer, III, has facilitated restoration of function and pain control in patients with a wide variety of shoulder problems. The advent of arthroscopy during the past decade has made many types of shoulder surgery possible without the morbidity associated with open surgery.

In most joint arthroplasties, patients are advised to use surgery as a last resort. The shoulder, however, is somewhat unique in that the soft tissues about the shoulder are critical for its function. Moreover, once end-stage disease occurs and motion is lost, it is difficult to restore that motion and function after total shoulder arthroplasty (TSA). Therefore, it is recommended that the patient with shoulder arthritis be referred to an orthopedic surgeon before end-stage disease develops. Therapy to increase and or maintain motion and rotator cuff strength should begin early in the progression of the disease. TSA should be considered before the rotator cuff is destroyed, the shoulder has proximally migrated, and the glenoid has eroded beyond the capacity to be resurfaced.

The purpose of this chapter is to acquaint physical therapists, occupational therapy practitioners, nurses, and orthopedic residents with shoulder surgery for rheumatic diseases and the role that integrated rehabilitation plays in the patient's recovery. This chapter reviews the biomechanics of the shoulder as they relate to function and surgery and the three most common rheumatic diseases that necessitate shoulder surgery:

1. rheumatoid arthritis (RA),
2. osteoarthritis (OA), and
3. osteonecrosis.

All of the surgical options are discussed, but the focus of the chapter will be on TSA because it requires the most planning and interdisciplinary teamwork of all shoulder procedures.

Shoulder Anatomy and Biomechanics

It is important to understand the surgical anatomy of the shoulder both for the diagnosis and management of shoulder arthritis. The glenohumeral joint is a shallow articulation designed to allow essentially universal motion of the shoulder joint. For this reason, the supporting structures are critical in maintaining the stability and enhanced function of shoulder articulation (Thornhill, 1994). The labrum of the shoulder joint as well as the capsular structures are stabilizers of the joint. The muscular activity about the shoulder is critical to stability. The rotator cuff is an important stabilizer of the humeral head as the powerful deltoid forward elevates and abducts the shoulder. The subscapularis acts as an internal rotator of the shoulder, and the other rotator cuff muscles (e.g., supraspinatus, infraspinatus, teres minor) act as external rotators. The external rotator cuff muscles attach to the greater tuberosity after moving through the subacromial space. This space is bounded superiorly by the undersurface of the acromion, inferiorly by the humeral head, and anteriorly by the coracoacromial ligament and coracoid process. Narrowing of this space or thickening tendinous structures may cause impingement leading to rotator cuff disease or pain (Neer, Craig, & Fukuda, 1983).

Pathophysiology

RA

The glenohumeral joint can be damaged by inflammatory arthritides such as RA and psoriatic arthritis and noninflammatory processes such as OA, posttraumatic arthritis, rotator cuff arthropathy, adhesive capsulitis, and avascular necrosis. Inflammatory processes involve a primary disease of the synovium, and noninflammatory processes involve a primary disease of the chondral surface. Their patterns of destruction can be quite different (Thornhill, 1993).

In RA, involvement of the glenohumeral joint is variable and is usually present in patients with progressive disease (Gordon & Hastings, 1994). The inflammatory process produces a synovitis with proliferation of cellular elements, which leads to destruction of the articular cartilage matrix. Articular cartilage is destroyed by a complex series of mechanisms that include activation of complement; release of cytokines, lymphokines, and growth factors; and production of superoxide-free radicals and other inflammatory components that amplify the inflammatory response (Schumacher, 1993).

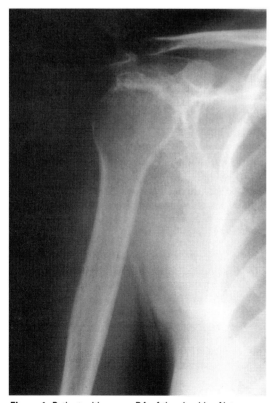

Figure 1. Patient with severe RA of the shoulder. Note erosion of humeral head and superior migration of the humerus, which indicates chronic rotator cuff tear.

The articular cartilage, unfortunately, is not the only target of the inflammatory process. The same mechanisms that destroy the joint surface damage the critical soft tissues of the shoulder. This may lead to subacromial bursitis and invasion and the eventual destruction of the rotator cuff (Kraay & Figgie, 1995). Moreover, pain makes it difficult to move, and not moving can lead to joint contracture and shortening of the subscapularis tendon. Destruction of the rotator cuff and loss of cuff function are frequently accompanied by proximal migration of the humeral head, which leads to a decrease of the subacromial space (Figure 1). It has been estimated that between 27% and 42% of patients with RA who have TSA have full-thickness rotator cuff tears (Kraay & Figgie, 1995). The typical radiographic appearance is one of joint-space narrowing and osteopenia without the typical sclerosis and osteophyte formation seen in noninflammatory conditions (Cofield, 1997).

OA

In noninflammatory joint disease, the pattern of destruction is different. Primary OA of the gleno-humeral joint is rare because the shoulder is normally not a weight-bearing joint and thus is less likely to sustain repeated heavy loads. In most cases, there is associated trauma, instability, or limited motion (e.g., adhesive capsulitis). Disorders that may create joint incongruity and lead to articular damage should be investigated if there is joint damage and no history of trauma. A neuropathic arthropathy could be caused by diabetes, syringomelia, or leprosy (Thornhill, 1993).

The radiographic pattern of OA is variable, but generally there is a major bony response with subchondral sclerosis and osteophyte formation. Involvement of the rotator cuff in noninflammatory joint disease is variable and often related to other associated problems such as longstanding impingement syndrome or a traumatic tear of the rotator cuff.

Impingement syndrome refers to acute or chronic impingement of the rotator cuff in the subacromial space. The etiology of this syndrome varies from repetitive overuse to congenital anatomical differences in the bony acromium (Neer et al., 1983). In the early and even chronic stages of

impingement syndrome, the glenohumeral joint is usually spared. In certain patients with end-stage impingement syndrome and disruption of the cuff, a proximal migration of the humerus occurs, leading to a condition known as *cuff tear arthropathy* (Neer et al., 1983). In cuff tear arthropathy, versus primary OA of the shoulder, proximal migration of the humeral head is always present, and joint destruction begins on the superior aspect of the humeral head (Figure 2). It is important to differentiate cuff tear arthropathy from other causes of shoulder pain because this problem can alter surgical outcome.

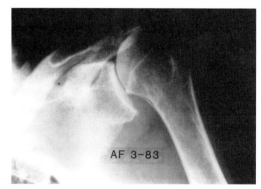

Figure 2. Patient with cuff arthropathy. Note debris and spur formation with misshapen humeral head.

Osteonecrosis

A humeral head fracture with or without fragment displacement (known as *avascular necrosis*) can be the precursor of osteonecrosis (Thornhill, 1993). This condition is cell death as a result of impairment of the blood supply to the humeral head (Mazieres, 1994). Steroid therapy for asthma, organ transplantation, sickle cell disease, systemic lupus erythematosus, or other systemic diseases can likewise lead to osteonecrosis (Figure 3).

Estimation of glenoid changes is critical in non-inflammatory joint disease because it substantially affects the choice of surgical procedures. In osteonecrosis, for instance, the glenoid may be

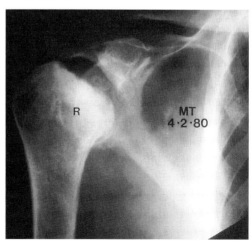

Figure 3. Osteonecrosis of the humeral head with associated collapse of the head and calcified debris.

totally spared. In primary OA, the glenoid may be anatomically normal with a smooth eburnated bony surface. In many cases, where there has been chronic instability and especially where an over-aggressive anterior capsular surgical procedure has been performed, there is posterior erosion of the glenoid and posterior subluxation of the humeral head (Boyd, Alibadi, & Thornhill, 1991; Boyd, Thomas, Scott, Sledge, & Thornhill, 1990).

Evaluation

A detailed history and physical examination will generally confirm the etiology of joint disease. A record of range of motion (ROM) and functional activity is essential both in determining the need for surgery and the results of that surgery. Patients typically reduce their ROM to avoid pain. A patient may function quite well with only 90° of shoulder flexion, but this can lead to marked joint contracture and increase the risk of OA. Although most TSAs reduce pain, the improvement in ROM is typically modest (Henry & Thornhill, 1994). This type of surgical intervention should be considered once it is clear that the joint is destroyed and limited ROM is related to functional loss.

Preoperative Considerations

Patients considering shoulder arthropathy often have other joint involvement and medical ailments, so it is important to evaluate these issues carefully preoperatively. The patient's general health and health-related behaviors (e.g., smoking, poor nutrition, diabetes, steroid use, vasculitis) may impede wound healing. The presence of osteoporosis may affect the choice of implant fixation. Certain arthritis medications will need to be altered in the perioperative period. In general, nonsteroidals are stopped a few days before surgery and are reinstituted postoperatively. Methotrexate is generally withheld in the perioperative period because changes in glomerular filtration rate and certain anti-infection medications may accentuate possible side effects.

It is important to evaluate the ipsilateral elbow and hand both in terms of positioning at surgery and during postoperative rehabilitation. Evaluation of neurological status must be carefully documented preoperatively. The patient's cervical spine must be evaluated both for stability and any evidence of cervical spondylosis, both of which will affect the choice of anesthesia and postoperative rehabilitation (Kraay & Figgie, 1995).

Imaging Studies

Radiographic evaluation should include a glenohumeral anteroposterior view in internal and external rotation as well as an axillary view. A scapular-Y view is valuable in evaluating trauma, but the axillary view is more important in evaluating the arthritic joint. Computed tomography (CT) and CT arthrography may be of great value in determining bony abnormalities of the glenoid and in estimating a need for bone grafting. Magnetic resonance imaging of the shoulder is less helpful for arthritis than it is in evaluating lesions of the rotator cuff in nonarthritic conditions. Magnetic resonance arthrography may enhance the diagnosis of labral pathology (i.e., damage to the labrum or fibro-cartilage ring around the glenoid cavity), but it has a limited role once arthritis has become established by plain radiographs (Thornhill, 1993).

Table 1. Simple Shoulder Test.

1. Do you think you can toss a softball underhand 10 yd. with the affected extremity?
2. Can you place a coin on the shelf at the level of your shoulder without bending your elbow?
3. Can you carry 20 lbs. (a bag of potatoes) at your side with the affected extremity?
4. Would your shoulder allow you to work full-time at your regular job?
5. Can you lift 8 lbs. (a full gallon container) to the level of the top of your head without bending your elbow?
6. Is your shoulder comfortable with your arm at rest by your side?
7. Does your shoulder allow you to sleep comfortably?
8. Can you reach the small of your back to tuck in your shirt with your hand?
9. Can you place your hand behind your head with the elbow straight out to the side?
10. Can you lift 1 lb. (a full pint container) to the level of your shoulder without bending your elbow?
11. Do you think you can throw a softball overhand 20 yd. with the affected extremity?
12. Can you wash the back of your opposite shoulder with the affected extremity?

Note. From *The shoulder: A balance of mobility and stability,* edited by F. A. Matsen and R. J. Hawkins, 1993, Rosemont, IL: American Academy of Orthopaedic Surgeons. Reprinted with permission.

Outcome Evaluation

Health status measures are essential in monitoring the effects of disease activity and in determining the outcome of interventions such as therapy and surgery. Both generic and disease-specific instruments are widely used in musculoskeletal conditions (Dorcas & Richard, 1996). The Medical Outcomes Study Short Form (SF-36; Ware & Sherbourne, 1992; see the appendix at the end of this book) is the most frequently used general health status instrument and has recently been used in a follow-up study of TSA (Matsen, 1996). Other functional assessments recommended are the Simple Shoulder Test (Table 1) and The Disabilities of the Shoulder Arm and Hand Instrument (DASH) developed by the Upper Extremity Collaborative Group (1996a, 1996b; Hudak, Amadio, Bombardier, & the Upper Extremity Collaborative Group, 1996; Lippitt, Harryman, & Matsen, 1993) (Appendix 1).

The orthopedist's office is probably the best place to collect the outcome data because of the routine follow-up that most surgeons endorse. Forms can either be mailed to the patient before the appointment, or the forms can be completed in the waiting area.

Conservative Management

Impingement syndromes and overuse syndromes of the rotator cuff are best treated with rest, activity modification, and anti-inflammatory medications. After the acute phase, exercises to restore motion and strength are begun with the goal of improving the biomechanics of the joint (Dalton, 1994). When there is articular disease, it is important to preserve, if not improve, motion. Modalities for pain relief with an emphasis on self-management are helpful as an adjunct to exercise, as are joint protection techniques. Ice is recommended for acute inflammation. For mild to moderate inflammation, many patients prefer heat. Both heat and cold modalities should be tried to determine which is more beneficial. Guidelines for activity modification with attention to repetitive tasks and static work positions and an ergonomic evaluation for patients employed in repetitive activities should be a part of the rehabilitation intervention. Intra-articular steroid injections may be helpful in controlling local synovitis and inflammation of periarticular structures, but they have not been found to offer as much relief in OA (Thornhill, 1993). No more than 2 to 4 injections per year are recommended, and when there is a need for more injections, alternative treatments are advised (Cofield, 1997; Schumacher, 1993).

Rehabilitation Evaluation

ROM and Strength

There is no consensus on which motions to record; however, elevation, external rotation, and internal rotation are the most critical to function. Whichever are chosen, the techniques should be standardized in the rehabilitation and orthopedic departments. Passive ROM should be measured. Lying down is more comfortable for patients with painful shoulders. The American Shoulder and Elbow Surgeons Society prefers elevation to flexion because more glenohumeral motion is possible when the humerus moves in elevation. Elevation is more functional than flexion.

Maximum elevation occurs when the long axis of the humerus lies in the plane of the scapula. This plane is approximately 45° to 60° from the coronal plane. "When glenohumeral motion is maximized in the elevation plane, scapulothoracic motion automatically allows maximum motion in the forward flexion and abduction planes" (Brems, 1994b). Trying to stretch or measure a patient's shoulder in a flexion plane is not accurate and will not be maximal because of the anatomical structure of the joint.

To record external rotation, a towel should be placed beneath the elbow, which should be brought away from the side to establish perpendicularity between the humerus and the glenoid. This will relax the capsule and allow for freer movement (Brems, 1994b). The greater tuberosity must externally rotate and clear the acromium, or elevation will not be possible, and there will be impingement. Loss of external rotation affects function because it is necessary for elevation.

Internal rotation is recorded by the spinal level or bony landmark that the tip of the thumb can reach (superior angle of the scapula = T4, inferior angle = T7, iliac crest = L4, gluteal crease = sacrum; reaching only posterior to the greater trochanter, anterior to the greater trochanter) (Greene & Heckman, 1994; Figure 4).

Recording ROM of the other joints with the exception of the contralateral shoulder is not time efficient, particularly if a functional evaluation is obtained. This is the same for strength testing, which is unreliable because of pain. Isometric testing, however, is helpful as an indication of the patient's ability to isolate muscle groups.

Preoperative Education

Preoperative education classes are uncommon for shoulder surgery. However, at the least, the patient should receive printed educational materials on the procedure and rehabilitation course. The orthopedic nurses in the clinic or surgeon's office should be knowledgeable in all aspects of the

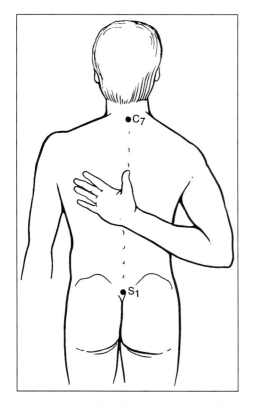

Figure 4. Posterior reach (internal rotation). Posterior reach essentially evaluates internal rotation of the shoulder with the arm at the side. This is a complex motion dependent on shoulder extension as well as elbow, wrist, and thumb motion. Posterior reach is defined as the highest midline segment of the back that is reached by the "hitch-hiking thumb." Most adults usually range from T6 to T10 spinous process. Young adults tend to reach higher, females to T4 and males to T5. Patients with arthritis of the shoulder and limited internal rotation may only be able to reach to the sacrum, gluteal region, greater trochanter, or lesser trochanter. *Note.* From *The clinical measurement of joint motion* (pp. 24–25), edited by W. B. Greene and J. D. Hechman, 1994, Rosemont, IL: American Academy of Orthopaedic Surgeons. Adapted with permission.

surgery and rehabilitation and should be available to discuss the patient's concerns and questions at a preoperative visit.

Discharge planning should begin before admission to the hospital. Home services or short-term admission to a skilled nursing facility may be needed for the patient who lives alone or who has polyarticular disease. For patients who have home supports, alternatives for tasks such as meal preparation, driving, and child care should be arranged. Assistance with activities of daily living (ADL) will be needed at least until the first postoperative visit, at which time precautions will be eased. Some patients believe that they can continue their independence immediately after the surgery. Arranging for assistance with ADL is essential and should be stressed because time must be available for exercising, and this cannot be done well if the joint and muscles are painful and fatigued.

Surgical Options

Arthroscopy

Although shoulder arthroscopy is helpful in evaluating and treating cuff disease, its use in shoulder arthritis is limited. Arthroscopic synovectomy may be quite helpful in decreasing pain and improving motion in the early stages of RA, when there is reasonable joint space and minimal joint destruction (Ellman & Gartsman, 1993). Arthroscopy may be a good diagnostic tool for a patient with monoarticular disease. In early noninflammatory joint disease, arthroscopy may be beneficial as a technique for efficient joint lavage, chondral debridement, and debridement of degenerative labral tears in the labrum or fibrocartilage ring around the glenoid cavity. Once there is major joint-space narrowing, however, arthroscopy has little role in the treatment of arthritis in the glenohumeral joint.

Acromioplasty

In some patients, RA or inflammatory arthritis weakens the rotator cuff so that the humeral head continually rides up and impinges on the acromion, which causes pain and further wear on the rotator cuff. Anatomical variations such as a hook-shaped acromion account for 70% of the split-thickness cuff tears (Bieber, 1994). Bone spurs on the inferior surface can damage the rotator cuff. Acromioplasty (i.e., the partial removal or shaping of the acromion) increases the subacromial space and can eliminate this impingement process. In RA, an acromioplasty is usually done in conjunction with a synovectomy or TSA.

Subacromial decompression can be performed either as an open or arthroscopic procedure. As an open procedure, the anterior portion of the acromion is removed along with the coracoacromial ligament. The subacromial bursa is excised, and the rotator cuff is examined and repaired if torn. This is done under direct visualization, and the arm is then placed in an elevated position to make sure that there is no further impingement. The undersurface of the acromioclavicular joint is carefully evaluated for any impingement at that point. Arthroscopically, subacromial decompression can be performed by first excising the subacromial bursa and then performing a subacromial decompression with an arthroscopic burr. The coracoacromial ligament can be divided by electrocautery and the rotator cuff examined. If there is a tear of the rotator cuff, a mini open procedure with direct suture of the cuff can be performed.

Postoperative Rehabilitation for Acromioplasty

Acromioplasty is usually performed in the day-surgery unit. If soft-tissue repair is done, it may necessitate a one-night hospital stay. Independent pendulum exercises and elbow, hand, and wrist movements are the usual recommendation until the first postoperative visit at 7 to 14 days. A sling is worn except when exercising and bathing. Some surgeons prearrange for a therapy appointment at the first follow-up visit. Instructions from the surgeon may be as simple as "progress motion and strength," with pain as the guiding factor. This requires teaching the basic rules for activity progression. Lifting is to be avoided for weeks as are overhead movements. The exercise focus is on strengthening the rotator cuff muscles and scapula stabilizers. The intensity of the rehabilitation will depend on the normal activities to which the patient must return.

Postoperative Rehabilitation for Nontraumatic Rotator Cuff Repair

Rotator cuff repair is most often done in conjunction with arthroscopic or TSA surgery. In most cases with articular involvement, a strengthening program is often initiated before surgery is considered in hopes of preventing the need for surgery because the outcome is less favorable.

Joint stability and soft-tissue healing are the aims of surgery, so the patient is immobilized in a sling and swathe for 6 weeks (Kraay & Figgie, 1995). Pendulum, elbow, and hand exercises are often performed the first day. Passive supine elevation may be allowed by the surgeon. When the soft tissue is sufficiently healed, the sling is discontinued, and the patient is encouraged to use the arm for

ADL. Increasing functional ROM is the goal. Isometric and resistive exercises are begun when tolerated by the patient.

Arthrodesis

Shoulder fusion is generally reserved for patients with neurological abnormalities about the shoulder such as a brachial plexus injury, chronic infection, and failed arthroplasties or in young, active patients whose activities will exceed those permitted with TSA (Cofield, 1997). The joint is usually fused in approximately 30° of abduction, flexion, and internal rotation and requires at least 6 weeks of immobilization in a thoracobrachial (airplane) orthosis. Gentle elbow and wrist ROM is recommended during the immobilization period (Richards, 1997). Richards, Sherman, Hudson, and Waddell (1988), in a review of 11 cases, found that all patients believed the surgery was beneficial and would have it again given the same circumstances. Eighty-two percent of the patients could feed and dress themselves, but they could not do work overhead. Long-term musculoskeletal consequences are not specifically addressed in the literature, but there tends to be increased scapulothoracic compensation, and there can be increased strain on the acromioclavicular joint.

Joint Arthroplasty

Joint replacement arthroplasty remains the mainstay for surgical treatment of the arthritic shoulder. Controversy remains about the role of hemiarthroplasty versus TSA for treatment of these disorders (Boyd et al., 1990). The data suggest that the choice of TSA or hemiarthroplasty depends on the etiology of the arthritis (Kraay & Figgie, 1995; Matsen, 1996; Neer, 1994). The major concern about TSA has been fixation of the glenoid component. A high incidence of glenoid loosening led many surgeons to choose hemiarthroplasty over TSA. Moreover, hemiarthroplasty is an easier operation to perform technically. The concern of hemiarthroplasty has been wear of the unresurfaced glenoid. Traditionally, articular cartilage, particularly in a damaged state, does not do well articulating with metal. Early wear of the cartilage and erosion of bone may occur. Moreover, pain relief may be incomplete.

TSA is indicated frequently in patients with RA, especially in those who have invasive pannus formation and bone erosion. In these cases, glenoid resurfacing can be combined with glenoid bone grafting in reestablishing glenoid bone stock and orientation of the glenoid surface.

Hemiarthroplasty is generally preferred in cases of osteonecrosis in which the glenoid is spared. It is likewise preferred in severe cuff tear arthropathy in which there is proximal migration of the humeral head. If the glenoid is resurfaced in these conditions, the proximal migration produces an eccentric load on the superior portion of the glenoid and facilitates loosening of the glenoid implant. Moreover, the proximal migration creates an incongruous articulation that promotes polyethylene wear. In noninflammatory joint disease, especially in younger active patients, hemiarthroplasty is preferred when the glenoid surface is smooth, even though there may be severe glenoid articular cartilage wear. Hemiarthroplasty is preferred in cases in which there is severe joint contracture, such as in juvenile rheumatoid arthritis. If one attempts to resurface the glenoid in these cases, there is a tendency to "overstuff" the joint, which leads to pain, limited motion, and increased joint reactive forces that promote wear.

Expectations and functional limitations. In general, patients are allowed to return to their usual ADL after a TSA. They are not allowed to participate in unlimited activity after surgery because of the concern of implant loosening and polyethylene wear. These limitations vary according to findings at surgery as well as the surgeon's philosophy. Repetitive activities above the level of the shoulder are frequently limited because of the preoperative condition of the rotator cuff. Repetitive lifting of objects greater than 25 lb is discouraged. Racket sports such as tennis, racquet ball, and squash are limited if not discouraged; the patient's desire to return to these activities would never be an indication for surgery. Recreational swimming with limited arm motion is permitted. Competitive jogging and other high-impact activities involving the lower extremities are discouraged because of the impact loading that occurs on the shoulder during these activities. Recreational golf with a modified swing is usually permitted; again, the desire to return to golf should never be an indication for surgery.

Patients who chronically bear weight through the upper extremity, for example, with crutch use and during wheelchair transfer have much greater shoulder pain (Williams & Iannotti, 1997). This is because of overuse of the soft tissue and stress on the acromioclavicular joint and glenoid cartilage. Activity modifications such as the use of a transfer board and crutch adaptations should be recommended before surgery. If crutch use is necessary, then axillary crutches should be recommended because some of the weight is distributed through the thorax instead of it all moving through the humeral head.

Surgical procedure and anesthesia. In most cases, regional anesthesia by interscalene block is preferred; most patients are given a supplemental general anesthetic for the procedure. In patients with RA, it is mandatory to evaluate the stability of the cervical spine, and, in many cases, fiber optic intubation is required. It will take several hours for the return of full sensation after an interscalene block (Friedman, 1994).

Exposure and implantation of a shoulder prosthesis can be technically demanding (Craig, 1995; Kraay & Figgie, 1995). The patient is positioned in a semireclining beach chair fashioned with a rolled towel behind the medial border of the scapula to improve glenoid exposure. A deltopectoral approach is generally preferred. The cephalic vein is spared if it can be retracted medially during the procedure. The coracoid is generally left intact, but, on occasion, a portion of the conjoined tendon may be released proximally to facilitate exposure and prevent traction on the musculocutaneous nerve. The vessels of the humeral circumflex vein are ligated and tied. They mark the inferior border of the subscapularis tendon and the level at which the axillary nerve courses anteriorly to innervate the deltoid. The upper portion of the subscapularis is identified by the long head of the biceps tendon that runs just superior to its upper edge. The subscapularis has a thickened upper edge that may be confused with the long head of the biceps. It is usually difficult to separate the subscapularis from the capsule, and these are frequently repaired as a single structure.

Subscapularis lengthening can be performed by separating the capsule and by blunt dissection to free adhesions above and below the muscle. Care must be taken to avoid injury to the axillary nerve, which can be palpated anteriorly and inferiorly to the subscapularis muscle. The shoulder is dislocated, and the humeral head is osteotomized in variable amounts of retroversion. In most cases where glenoid anatomy is normal, the humerus is osteotomized in 40° to 45° of retroversion. If there is retroversion of the glenoid that cannot be corrected, it is frequently necessary to place less humeral

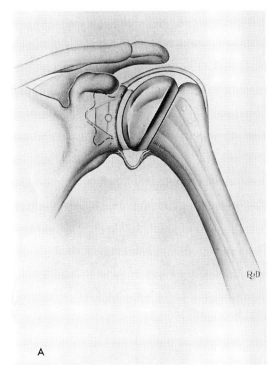 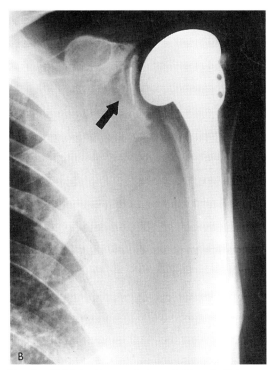

Figure 5. The illustration (A) and the X-ray film (B) show the standard long head total shoulder resurfacing unit. The polyethylene glenoid component is anchored with acrylic cement *(arrow)*. The metal humeral head has an intramedullary fixation stem, which does not require cement. The humeral stem is available in three diameters and lengths. (From Neer, C.S., II. Used with permission.)

retroversion to prevent posterior subluxation of the humeral head. The glenoid is exposed with a retractor placed posteriorly and anteriorly to the glenoid. The glenoid vault is entered with a burr and outlined with a curved curette. The long axis of the glenoid vault runs anteriorly in its superior portion and somewhat posteriorly in the inferior portion. It acts as fixation for the keel of the glenoid component and for determining the orentation of the glenoid surface. If the keel of the trial implant is placed in the prepared vault, and there is no contact posteriorly, this suggests posterior erosion of the glenoid and the need for a posterior glenoid graft. In most cases, the surgeon author (T.S.T.) prefers an uncemented glenoid componenet fixed with two screws. If rigid fixation cannot be obtained, an all-polyethylene glenoid is cemented after the canal has been carefully prepared and the cement pressurized. The humeral component is usually uncemented when rigid press-fit fixation can be achieved during the operation and the implant is resistant to rotation. In cases of marked proximal humeral destruction or in severe osteopenia, it is necessary to cement the humerl component (Figure 5).

The subscapularis is carefully repaired. The rotator cuff is inspected and repaired. Proximal placement of the subscapularis tendon can facilitate cuff repair and act as a humeral depresser during motion. After repair of the subscapularis and the rotatttor cuff, the shoulder is carried through the ranges of forward elevation, internal rotation, external rotation, and abduction to determine the anatomical ROM possible, when unlimited by pain, to guide postoperative rehabilitation. The integrity of the cuff repair is estimated to determine how aggressive the postoperative program will be. If the anterior deltoid muscle is released for exposure, this must be conveyed to the rehabilitation team so that active forward elevation is limited in the early postoperative period. In cases of severe, irreparable rotator cuff tear, hemiarthroplasty is performed primarily for pain relief, for without the cuff there is no stability in the shoulder (Figure 6).

Rehabilitation protocols. The average hospitalization for a TSA is 3 to 5 days. To individualize the rehabilitation protocol, the practitioner must know several preoperative and perioperative variables. These include:

- preoperative ROM and function,
- method of exposure (whether the deltoid is released),
- the integrity of the subscapularis repair,
- the status of the rotator cuff,
- interoperative ROM and stability of the fixation,
- the surgeon's goals for the patient, and
- patient-specific postoperative precautions.

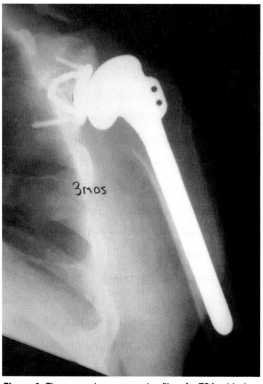

Figure 6. Three-month postoperative film of a TSA with the glenoid component anchored with screws.

In the 1970s, Hughes and Neer (1975) described the first protocol for rehabilitation of the modern glenohumeral joint replacement. These guidelines have been altered over the years to reflect surgical improvements and reduced the length of hospitalization. When these guidelines were developed, the patient was hospitalized for 14 days. Neer's original guidelines described three phases and date of initiation:

- Phase I: assisted ROM and isometrics (0–14 days)
- Phase II: active exercises and strengthening (4–6 weeks)
- Phase III: vigorous stretching (more than 6 weeks)

There are numerous published protocols indicating that there is no agreement on which protocol is best. Brems (1994a, 1994b) described a mobilizations phase, a stretching phase, and a strengthening phase, each with subsets. All exercise sessions should be brief and last about 5 min. Motion and stretching should be done 3 to 5 times a day and strengthening once a day.

Evaluation of neurovascular status and wound and skin integrity. It will take several hours for the return of full sensation after interscalene or axillary blocks. Neurovascular checks are completed by nursing staff members every 2 to 4 hr, and compromises are reported to the surgeon. The surgeon will set a parameter for hemovac output if one is used, and the surgeon should be notified if it is exceeded. Drainage on the dressing, which more likely will be found on the posterior aspect of the upper arm and elbow rather than directly over the incision, should be noted. After the initial dressing change by the surgeon, which is usually on postoperative day (POD) 1, nursing staff members gently wash the surgical arm. Care must be taken when removing the sling and abducting the arm to wash and dry the axilla. Powder is not used, but soft dressing material is placed in the axilla to absorb perspiration and prevent skin breakdown. The pad is changed twice daily, and the arm and incision are inspected for swelling and signs of skin breakdown or infection.

Pain management. The patient's perception of pain character and intensity should be recorded with a 0 to 10 analog scale. Patient-controlled anesthesia is an effective method of pain management for the first 24 to 48 hr. Oral pain medications are usually administered after the second day. During the hospitalization, the patient is encouraged to take medication 30 min before therapy and at bed time if sleeping is affected.

Postoperative positioning. Proper positioning is essential to prevent dislocation, to minimize tension on the incision site, and to minimize muscle spasm and pain in the neck, back, and shoulders. The patient's arm will be positioned by the surgeon, usually in a sling and swathe dressing. The head of the bed should be elevated at least 30°, and a pillow, pad, or folded blanket should be placed to support the humerus in alignment with the glenoid (Figure 7). The hand is elevated to minimize swelling. An abduction airplane splint may be used after rotator cuff repair. Compliance with the use of the immobilizer sling and with movement restrictions should be enforced during hospitalization. If the restrictions are to continue at discharge, their rationale should be discussed with the patient to ensure compliance.

In the initial postoperative period, the patient will need assistance with bathing, toileting, eating, and most other ADL. Self-care activities will feel awkward and difficult because of the restrictions on the operative arm. As motion is allowed and strength increases, the patient should be encouraged to move within the limits of pain. All important objects such as the telephone, water, and utensils should be within reach of the other arm.

Deep breathing, coughing, and moving in bed is recommended every 2 hr during the first 24-hr period to prevent respiratory complications. Antiembolism stockings should be worn until the patient is ambulating, and ankle-pump exercises should be encouraged during waking hours. Other joints should have active or assisted ROM to prevent stiffness. Cervical ROM is encouraged, and the patient is allowed to have his or her own pillow brought into the hospital after surgery. On POD 1, most patients will require assistance with transfers and ambulation. The affected arm will feel heavier, and balance will be altered, especially if the affected arm is the dominant arm.

Exercises for the hand and wrist should begin before the primary dressing is changed and the hemovac is removed. Retrograde massage of the fingers and forearm can be taught to the patient. Compressive wrapping with Coban™ (3M, St. Paul, MN) from the digits to the elbow may help

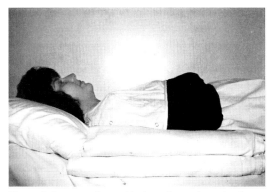

Figure 7. Postoperative positioning: sling and swathe dressing, head of the bed elevated 30°, pads or blankets to support the humerus in alignment with the glenoid, and the hand elevated to reduce swelling.

reduce the edema. Once the incision has been checked by the surgeon, shoulder motion can begin according to protocol, and precautions should be discussed with the patient. Stiffness and pain are expected but can be controlled by having frequent short sessions of exercise and by establishing a medication schedule.

Precautions (4–6 weeks or at the surgeon's discretion).

- External rotation in adduction only to neutral to protect subscapularis repair
- Abduction (if allowed) in neutral or internal rotation
- Internal rotation in adduction only
- No resistive exercises (light ADL [hand-to-mouth tasks] are permitted)
- Nighttime sling and swathe to limit external rotation

Postoperative exercise program. The following exercise progression is a combination of the Brigham and Women's Hospital (Boston, MA) protocol and that of other published guidelines (Craig, 1995; Hughes & Neer, 1975; Matsen, 1996) (Appendix 2 for a sample progressive exercise program).

Exercises are begun in supine with the arm supported and in slight abduction. This position will lessen pain and compensatory scapular motion. Assistance is given to elbow flexion and extension, internal rotation from the chest toward neutral, and shoulder elevation. Pain and swelling will be minimized if the practitioner is not overzealous on the first day. Patients are involved in therapy from the start, when they are taught to do active and active assisted ROM. Three to five short sessions of less than 10 repetitions each are recommended per day (Brems, 1994a, 1994b). (See Appendices 2 and 3 for samples of inpatient and home programs. Instructions in precautions and rationale for progression are discussed on POD 1.)

If allowed, gradual weaning from the sling during the day begins on POD 2. Forward elevation is critical to function. Exercising with the elbow bent (shorter lever arm of force) requires less strength and tension across the shoulder joint. It is additionally a method for the patient to gauge progress. Reaching landmarks (e.g., mouth, nose, forehead, pillow) can be motivating to the patient. Active elevation in this manner adheres to the internal rotation restrictions and facilitates light ADL. Assistance from the other arm is encouraged, and family members are instructed in exercise techniques.

The limit of elevation in the early postoperative phase is determined by the interoperative measurements and the patient's level of comfort. Patients report more pain with lowering the arm than with raising the arm. Instruction to "lightly push" the posterior humerus into the practitioner's hand or the patient's other hand, instead of just lowering, will stabilize the joint and lessen the pain.

Abduction is not emphasized in early rehabilitation, and active abduction is definitely not permitted if there has been a repair to the supraspinatus tendon. If assisted motion is permitted, the patient would begin by simply sliding the hand from the stomach across the pelvis to the hip. This maintains the shoulder in internal rotation.

The motion is progressed during the 3 to 5 days of hospitalization, at which time the patient spends more time out of the sling and is encouraged to relax and lightly swing the arm during ambulation. As with exercise, frequent short sessions out of the sling are recommended. The arm should be supported when it becomes tired or painful. The sling is worn at night for 4 to 6 weeks. It should be worn out in public as a "red flag" to caution others.

Assisted exercise techniques vary. Continuous passive motion (CPM) machines are available for the shoulder in supine and sitting positions but can be difficult to set up (Craig, 1986). A CPM machine may be of benefit when the patient is unable to assist in the exercise program, but there can be safety issues if there has been extensive soft-tissue repair. If CPM is begun on the day of surgery, heavier wound drainage should be expected (Johnson, 1993).

Pendulum and pulley exercises are assisted exercises that must be sanctioned by the surgeon before initiating. For pulley exercises, the patient should initially sit facing the pulley. The instruction is to pull the arm forward and up with the unoperated side. Later in the program, when there is a smooth 90° of elevation, the patient can stand or sit with his or her back to the pulley for a greater stretch. Technique and form during this exercise is important because the intent is to increase glenohumeral motion, not scapulothoracic motion.

Isometric exercises, if allowed, are begun usually after discharge from the hospital but before the first follow-up visit. If the patient will not be receiving outpatient or home therapy, the exercise should be taught in the hospital but practiced on the nonoperated side. Light contraction and no motion should be emphasized.

Applications of lightweight cold compresses are suggested for swelling and pain relief. Hot packs for relaxation of muscles before exercise are used in some facilities (Brems, 1994a, 1994b) but should not be placed directly over the incision because heat applied early in wound healing can increase fibrinogen release, which in turn can increase scar formation (Hardy, 1989).

ADL. As soon as motion has begun, the patient is encouraged to participate in light self-care activities in adduction such as eating and dressing. The patient should be instructed to dress the operated side first to avoid abduction and external rotation and to write in the midline position instead of in external rotation beyond neutral. Showering begins at the surgeon's discretion. The patient must be able to get the sling on and off easily and safely. A sling with sturdy Velcro® closures will eliminate the need for adaptation. If the expectation is that the patient will achieve greater than 90° of elevation, adaptive equipment with extended handles for reaching, grooming, and so forth is not indicated. It is important to consider the nonoperated extremity as well as hand dominance when evaluating equipment needs. Devices with extended handles create a long lever arm, which increases the force on the hand, shoulder, and elbow joints.

Discharge planning. Discharge plans begin on POD 1 if they have not been discussed before surgery. Precautions and exercise instructions must be discussed with the caregivers, particularly if they will be assisting with the exercise program (see Appendices 1 and 3). Some physicians prefer that patients implement their own program or only receive therapy from the surgical facility because of the limited experience with TSA in most community and home health care practices. It is the responsibility of the inpatient practitioner to educate the community practitioner and guide the home program. The patient should be given a list of the precautions and the exercise progression guidelines for his or her next practitioner. Calling the local practitioner and sending him or her the surgical report is recommended.

Program advancement. The first postoperative surgical visit is usually 4 to 6 weeks after the operation (unless sutures must be removed). Exercises are progressed, and activity precautions are usually revised if not eliminated. (See Appendix 2 in this chapter.) If the patient has been doing an independent home program, then it is recommended that an outpatient therapy appointment be scheduled so that the exercise program can be advanced. If the patient is receiving home or community therapy, the surgeon should provide updated instruction.

In general, external rotation, internal rotation, and abduction are allowed as tolerated, and assisted motions can be progressed to active motion. Controlled stretching with attention to scapula motion can begin. Motion should be maximized before strengthening becomes the focus of the rehabilitation. Interoperative motions should not be exceeded because this can lead to failure from stretching the soft tissue. Combined stretches such as elevation with abduction and external rotation and internal rotation with extension are useful in functional activities. Patients with OA or those who have had a TSA secondary to a fracture usually progress faster and may be allowed to do these stretches in the first few weeks (Brems, 1994a, 1994b).

Aquatic exercise for persons with arthritis is excellent because buoyancy can both assist a motion and offer resistance for strengthening, and combined functional motions can be practiced with less fatigue (Sova, 1992). Exercising in water before the surgical precautions are lifted should be done cautiously. The patient may not be able to control the effects of buoyancy, thus stressing soft-tissue repair. Water is a difficult medium in which to control scapulothoracic movement. If the patient is to begin or resume aquatic exercise after the precautions have been removed, it is advised that he or she receive instruction from a water therapy practitioner who can modify the program on the basis of knowledge of the physical properties of water as an exercise medium.

Theraband™ (Hygenic Corp., Akron, OH) is often recommended by surgeons for strengthening because it is lightweight, portable, inexpensive, and available in varying degrees of resistance. Theraband™ requires greater tension because the muscle is shortened and moved through its arc of motion. This is contrary to the principles of the length–tension relationship and the effects of the joint angle on the ability of a muscle to produce tension (Hamill & Knutzen, 1995). A muscle has a reduced mechanical advantage at the extremes of range, and the patient must be aware of this concept and exercise with caution. Before dispensing the Theraband™, the patient's sensitivity or allergy to latex materials should be determined. Patients with RA may find it more comfortable to loop the Theraband™ around the wrist. (See Appendix 3 in this chapter.)

Strengthening exercises for the scapula-stabilizing muscles are essential to glenohumeral motion and function and can be done with Theraband™ or weights. Whichever form is used, scapulothoracic substitution should be prevented; it tends to occur when there is insufficient glenohumeral motion or the weight or band is too heavy. Figure 8 depicts a hemiarthroplasty patient doing active flexion and exercising with a free weight in supine position. Note the difference in compensatory movement. This patient should work on achieving greater control in supine position before progressing to exercises in the sitting or standing positions.

A strengthening protocol from the Cleveland Clinic (Cleveland, OH) consists of three strengthening phases (Brems, 1994a, 1994b):

- Phase I exercises are done in the supine position, which minimizes the effect of gravity. The emphasis is on glenohumeral control from 0 to 90° of elevation and eccentrically controlling

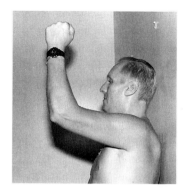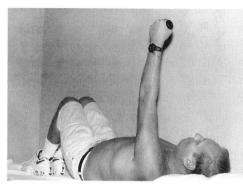

Figure 8. (A left): Patient in postoperative outpatient therapy after a hemiarthroplasty for osteonecrosis. Note the scapulothoracic substitution on the left during active flexion. (B right): Patient is able to strengthen muscles without scapula compensation.

the motion as the arm is lowered to 0°. When 10 repetitions without pain are possible, then weight is added and increased by 0.5 lb. Forces on the hand, wrist, and elbow must be considered when weights are used in any position. Cuff weights are preferable to hand-held weights for patients with hand or wrist pain and weakness.

- Phase II is eccentric strengthening in sitting or standing position. The arm can be assisted to its maximum range, and the deceleration is controlled as the arm is lowered. Weight is slowly added when 10 repetitions can be done without fatigue. The weight is increased in 0.5-lb increments.

- Phase III is strengthening for the anterior, middle, and posterior deltoid and the individual cuff muscles. Many patients will not progress beyond the light resistance bands of yellow or red. They should, however, try to increase the number of repetitions and the duration that each contraction is held. The scapula stabilizers, especially the serratus anterior and rhomboids, will need strengthening. Strength gains can be slow, and maximum benefit may not be seen for 6 months to 1 year. Formal therapy should continue for at least 6 to 8 weeks but preferably as long as functional goals are being achieved. Because many insurance plans do not cover long-term therapy, each patient should have a written outline of how to independently progress the exercise program.

Outcomes. Most TSAs performed at the Robert Breck Brigham Hospital (Boston, MA) and later at Brigham and Women's Hospital have been of the Neer series (Barrett, Franklin, Jackins, Wyss, & Matsen, 1987; Friedman, Thornhill, Thomas, & Sledge, 1989). In most cases, the humeral component is press-fit, although, in approximately 30% of cases, it is necessary to cement the humeral component. In the initial series, glenoid resurfacing was performed with a polyethylene-cemented component. For a short time, a metal-backed cemented glenoid was used, but in recent years an uncemented press-fit and screw-fixed glenoid has been preferred when the glenoid component is resurfaced. In most reported series, pain relief after TSA has been greater than 91% (Barrett et al., 1987; Figgie et al., 1988; Friedman et al., 1989). Patients with RA and OA had an improvement in postoperative forward elevation compared with the preoperative level. Persons with OA, however, had better forward elevation overall and gained more forward elevation compared with those with RA (Cofield, 1997). The most important factor determining postoperative forward elevation is preoperative forward elevation and the ability to restore rotator cuff function. By using a series of functional activity questions, both patients with RA and OA had a major increase in their postoperative function, and that gain in functional activity seemed to be maintained during the period of postoperative evaluation. By comparing patients with RA and

OA, the results were equivalent in terms of pain relief, functional score, and the patient's evaluation of the procedure (Cofield, 1997).

Complications. From the literature, on the basis of Neer-type implants, Cofield (1997) tabulated the complications for 1,459 TSAs. Overall complication rate was 14%, with 5.2% having glenohumeral instability and 1.9% having glenoid loosening. In the Boyd and colleagues (1991) series, 12% of the components showed evidence of component migration, and 6% required revision at 4 to 7 years postoperatively. Use of a metal-backed cemented glenoid did not improve these data, and, in fact, the stiff metal backing may facilitate polyethylene wear. Current recommendations are to use an all-polyethylene component when the glenoid is cemented. Humeral loosening was rare.

Other complications include dislocation, axillary nerve palsy, greater tuberosity fracture, rotator cuff tear, and infection, which occurs in 0.5% of cases (Cofield, 1996; Laurence, 1991). In cases of dislocation or subluxation, it is often noted that there is an associated component malposition. Fracture after TSA most likely will occur in the mid-portion of the humerus distal to the implant. If the fracture can be well aligned and stabilized during joint motion, a nonoperative treatment is preferred. In cases in which the fracture cannot be stabilized during joint motion or when evidence of callus formation does not appear within a few weeks, it is necessary to perform open reduction and internal fixation. In some cases, it is necessary to revise the humeral component to a longer intramedullary stem to achieve fracture fixation.

Summary

Treating the cuff-deficient shoulder is still a major problem. In these patients, hemiarthroplasty is preferred. Proximal migration with impingement into the subacromial space and the coracoacromial arch is the rule rather than the exception. Bipolar hemiarthroplasty, surface hemiarthroplasty, massive cuff repair, occluded glenoids, and even subacromial bumpers have been used to prevent this problem. To date, there is no effective, predictable method to perform TSA in patients with massive rotator cuff tears and proximal migration.

The major problem with TSA is wear and stability. The bearing surfaces of metal and polyethylene will produce wear debris that may cause osteolysis. This does not seem to be as great a problem in the shoulder as in the hip. As better materials with less wear-debris production are developed, the longevity of shoulder implants will be enhanced.

It is essential that clinic nurses and practitioners continually monitor the function of the patients' shoulders and instruct them in a program that will help maintain motion and strength. This should occur even before the patient reports difficulties with ADL that may not be evident until considerable ROM is lost. Joint protection techniques to decrease the forces across the glenohumeral surfaces should likewise be advised.

References

Barrett, W. P., Franklin, J. L., Jackins, S. E., Wyss, C. R., & Matsen F. A. (1987). Total shoulder arthroplasty. *Journal of Bone and Joint Surgery 69A*, 865–872.

Bieber, E. J. (1994). Orthopedic management of the shoulder in rheumatic disease. In J. H. Klippel & P. A. Dieppe (Eds.), *Rheumatology* (pp. 8-21.1–8-21.6). St. Louis, MO: Mosby.

Boyd, A. D., Alibadi, P., & Thornhill, T. S. (1991). Postoperative proximal migration in total shoulder arthroplasty: Incidence and significance. *Journal of Arthroplasty, 6,* 31–37.

Boyd, A. D., Thomas, W. H., Scott, R. D., Sledge, C. B., & Thornhill, T. S. (1990). Total shoulder arthroplasty versus hemiarthroplasty: Indications for glenoid surfacing. *Journal of Arthroplasty, 5,* 329–336.

Brems, J. J. (1994a). Rehabilitation following shoulder arthroplasty. In R. H. Friedman (Ed.), *Arthroplasty of the shoulder* (pp. 99–112). New York: Thieme Medical.

Brems, J. J. (1994b). Rehabilitation following total shoulder arthroplasty. *Clinical Orthopedics and Related Research, 307,* 70–85.

Cofield, R. H. (1996). Results and complications of shoulder arthroplasty. In B. Morrey (Ed.), *Reconstructive surgery of the joints* (pp. 773–788). New York: Churchill Livingstone.

Cofield, R. H. (1997). The shoulder. In W. N. Kelley, E. D. Harris, S. Ruddy, & C. B. Sledge (Eds.), *Textbook of rheumatology* (pp. 1696–1712). Philadelphia: Saunders.

Craig, E. (1986). Continuous passive motion after shoulder reconstruction. *Orthopedic Transcripts, 10,* 219.

Craig, E. V. (1995). *Kirschner integrated shoulder system for hemi and total shoulder arthroplasty: Surgical technique.* Hunt Valley, MD: Kirschner Medical.

Dalton, S. E. (1994). The shoulder. In J. H. Klippel & P. A. Dieppe (Eds.), *Rheumatology* (5-8.1–5-8.16). St Louis, MO: Mosby.

Dorcas, E. B., & Richard, R. R. (1996). Measuring function in shoulders. *Journal of Bone and Joint Surgery, 78A,* 882–889.

Ellman, H. & Gartsman, G. M. (Eds.). (1993). Glenohumeral arthritis. *Arthroscopic shoulder surgery and related procedures* (pp. 317–332). Philadelphia: Lea & Febiger.

Figgie, H. E. III, Inglis, A. E., Goldberg, V. M., Ranawat, C. S., Figgie, M. P., & Wile, J. M. (1988). An analysis of factors affecting the long-term results of total shoulder arthroplasty in inflammatory arthritis. *Journal of Arthroplasty, 3,* 123.

Friedman, R. J., Thornhill, T. S., Thomas, W. H., & Sledge, C. B. (1989). Non-constrained total shoulder replacements in patients who have rheumatoid arthritis and class IV function. *Journal of Bone and Joint Surgery, 71A,* 494–498.

Gordon, D. A., & Hastings, D. E. (1994). Clinical features: Early, progressive and late disease. In J. H. Klippel & P. A. Dieppe (Eds.), *Rheumatology* (pp. 3-4.1–4-14). St. Louis, MO: Mosby.

Greene, W. B., & Heckman, J. D. (Eds.). (1994). *The clinical measurement of joint motion.* Rosemont, IL: American Academy of Orthopedic Surgeons.

Hamill, J., & Knutzen, K. M. (Eds.). (1995). *Biomechanical basic of human movement.* Media, PA: Williams & Wilkins.

Hardy, M. A. (1989). The biology of scar formation. *Physical Therapy, 69,* 1014–1024.

Henry, J. D., & Thornhill, T. S. (1994). Long term results of total shoulder arthroplasty. In R. J. Friedman (Ed.), *Arthroplasty of the shoulder* (pp. 227–233). New York: Thieme Medical.

Hudak, P. I., Amadio, P. C., Bombardier, C., & the Upper Extremity Collaborative Group. (1996). Development of an upper extremity outcome measure: The DASH (Disability of the Arm, Shoulder and Hand). *American Journal of Industrial Medicine, 29,* 602–608.

Hughes, M., & Neer, C. S. (1975). Glenohumeral joint replacement and postoperative rehabilitation. *Physical Therapy, 55,* 850–858.

Johnson, R. L. (1993). Total shoulder arthroplasty. *Orthopedic Nursing, 12*, 14–22.

Kraay, M. J., & Figgie, M. P. (1995). The shoulder. In T. P. Sculco (Ed.), *Surgical treatment of rheumatoid arthritis* (pp. 127–145). St Louis, MO: Mosby-Year Book.

Laurence, M. (1991). Replacement arthroplasty of the rotator cuff deficient shoulder. *Journal of Bone and Joint Surgery, 73B*, 916–919.

Lippitt, S. B., Harryman, D. T., & Matsen, F. A. (1993). A practical tool for evaluation of function: The simple shoulder test. In F. A. Matsen & R. J. Hawkins (Eds.), *The shoulder: A balance of mobility and stability* (pp. 8–15). Rosemont, IL: American Academy of Orthopedic Surgeons.

Matsen, F. A. (1996). Early effectiveness of shoulder arthroplasty for patients who have primary degenerative disease. *Journal of Bone and Joint Surgery, 78A*, 260–264.

Mazieres, B. (1994). Osteonecrosis. In J. H. Klippel & P. A. Dieppe (Eds.), *Rheumatology* (pp. 7.41.1–7.41.8). St Louis, MO: Mosby.

Neer, C. S. (1994). Surgery in the shoulder. In W. H. Kelly, E. D. Harris, S. Ruddy, & C. B. Sledge (Eds.), *Surgery in arthritis* (pp. 754–769). Philadelphia: Saunders.

Neer, C. S., Craig, E. V., & Fukuda, H. (1983). Cuff tear arthropathy. *Journal of Bone and Joint Surgery, 65A*, 1232–1244.

Richards, R. R. (1997). Redefining indications and problems of shoulder arthrodesis. In J. J. P. Warner, J. B. Iannotti, & C. Gerber (Eds.), *Complex and revision problems in shoulder surgery* (pp. 319–338). Philadelphia: Lippincott-Raven.

Richards, R., Sherman, R., Hudson, A., & Waddell, J. (1988). Shoulder arthrodesis using a pelvic-reconstruction plate: A report of eleven cases. *Journal of Bone and Joint Surgery, 70A*, 416–421.

Schumacher, H. R. (Ed.). (1993). *Primer on the rheumatic diseases*. Atlanta, GA: Arthritis Foundation.

Sova, R. (1992). *Aquatics: The complete reference guide for aquatic fitness professionals*. Boston: Jones & Bartlett.

Thornhill, T. S. (1993). Shoulder pain. In W. N. Kelley, E. D. Harris, S. Ruddy, & C. B. Sledge (Eds.), *Textbook of rheumatology* (pp. 413–440). Philadelphia: Saunders.

Thornhill, T. S. (1994). Shoulder pain. In W. N. Kelley, E. D. Harris, C. B. Sledge, & S. Ruddy (Eds.), *Arthritis surgery* (pp. 201–224). Philadelphia: Saunders.

Upper Extremity Collaborative Group. (1996a). Development of an upper extremity outcome measure: The DASH (Disability of the Arm, Shoulder, and Hand). *Arthritis and Rheumatism, 39*(9), S112.

Upper Extremity Collaborative Group. (1996b). Measuring disability and symptoms of the upper limb: A validation study of the DASH questionnaire. *Arthritis and Rheumatism, 39*(9), S112.

Ware, J., & Sherbourne, C. (1992). The MOS 36 item short form health survey (SF-36). *Medical Care, 30*, 473–482.

Williams, G. R., & Iannotti, J. B. (1997). The weight-bearing shoulder. In J. P. Warner, J. B. Iannotti, & C. Gerber (Eds.), *Complex and revision problems in shoulder surgery* (pp. 2-03-2-12). Philadelphia: Lippincott-Raven.

Appendix 1
The Disabilities of the Arm, Shoulder, and Hand Instrument (DASH)

> **INSTRUCTIONS:** This questionnaire asks about your symptoms as well as your ability to perform certain activities.
>
> Please answer **every question**, based on your condition in the last week, by circling the appropriate number.
>
> If you did not have the opportunity to perform an activity in the past week, please make your **best guess** as to which response would be the most accurate.
>
> It doesn't matter which hand or arm you use to perform the activity; please answer based on your ability regardless of how you perform the task.

PART A

Please rate your ability to do the following activities in the last week by circling the number in the box below the appropriate response.

	NO DIFFICULTY	MILD DIFFICULTY	MODERATE DIFFICULTY	SEVERE DIFFICULTY	UNABLE
1. Open a tight or new jar.	1	2	3	4	5
2. Write.	1	2	3	4	5
3. Turn a key.	1	2	3	4	5
4. Prepare a meal.	1	2	3	4	5
5. Push open a heavy door.	1	2	3	4	5
6. Place an object on a shelf above your head.	1	2	3	4	5
7. Do heavy household chores (e.g., wash walls, wash floors).	1	2	3	4	5
8. Garden or do yardwork.	1	2	3	4	5
9. Make a bed.	1	2	3	4	5
10. Carry a shopping bag or briefcase.	1	2	3	4	5
11. Carry a heavy object (over 10 lb.)	1	2	3	4	5

Appendix 1 (cont.)

12. Change a lightbulb overhead.	1	2	3	4	5
13. Wash or blow dry your hair.	1	2	3	4	5
14. Wash your back.	1	2	3	4	5
15. Put on a pullover sweater.	1	2	3	4	5
16. Use a knife to cut food.	1	2	3	4	5
17. Recreational activities that require little effort (e.g., cardplaying, knitting).	1	2	3	4	5
18. Recreational activities in which you take some force or impact through your arm, shoulder, or hand (e.g., golf, hammering, tennis).	1	2	3	4	5
19. Recreational activities in which you move your arm freely (e.g., playing frisbee, badminton).	1	2	3	4	5
20. Manage transportation needs (getting from one place to another).	1	2	3	4	5
21. Sexual activities.	1	2	3	4	5

22. During the past week, **to what extent** has your arm, shoulder, or hand problem interfered with your normal social activities with family, friends, neighbors, or groups? (*circle number*)

NOT AT ALL	SLIGHTLY	MODERATELY	QUITE A BIT	EXTREMELY
1	2	3	4	5

23. During the past week, were you limited in your work or other regular daily activities as a result of your arm, shoulder, or hand problem? (*circle numbers*)

NOT LIMITED AT ALL	SLIGHTLY LIMITED	MODERATELY LIMITED	VERY LIMITED	UNABLE
1	2	3	4	5

Appendix 1 (cont.)

PART B

Please rate the severity of the following symptoms in the last week. (*circle number*)

	NONE	MILD	MODERATE	SEVERE	EXTREME
24. Arm, shoulder, or hand pain.	1	2	3	4	5
25. Arm, shoulder, or hand pain when you performed any specific activity.	1	2	3	4	5
26. Tingling (pins and needles) in your arm, shoulder, or hand.	1	2	3	4	5
27. Weakness in your arm, shoulder, or hand.	1	2	3	4	5
28. Stiffness in your arm, shoulder, or hand.	1	2	3	4	5

29. During the past week, how much difficulty have you had sleeping because of the pain in your arm, shoulder, or hand? (*circle number*)

NO DIFFICULTY	MILD DIFFICULTY	MODERATE DIFFICULTY	SEVERE DIFFICULTY	SO MUCH DIFFICULTY THAT I CAN'T SLEEP
1	2	3	4	5

30. I feel less capable, less confident, or less useful because of my arm, shoulder, or hand problem. (*circle number*)

STRONGLY DISAGREE	DISAGREE	NEITHER AGREE NOR DISAGREE	AGREE	STRONGLY AGREE
1	2	3	4	5

PART C—SPORTS/PERFORMING ARTS (OPTIONAL)

The following questions relate to the impact of your arm, shoulder, or hand problem on playing **your musical instrument or sport or both.**

If you play more than one sport or instrument (or play both), please answer with respect to that activity that is most important to you.

Please indicate the sport or instrument that is most important to you: _____

Appendix 1 (cont.)

Please circle the number that best describes your physical ability in the past week. Did you have any difficulty?

	NO DIFFICULTY	MILD DIFFICULTY	MODERATE DIFFICULTY	SEVERE DIFFICULTY	UNABLE
1. Using your usual technique for playing your instrument or sport?	1	2	3	4	5
2. Playing your musical instrument or sport because of arm, shoulder, or hand pain?	1	2	3	4	5
3. Playing your muscial instrument or sport as well as you would like?	1	2	3	4	5
4. Spending your usual amount of time practicing or playing your instrument or sport?	1	2	3	4	5

Scoring the DASH

The DASH is scored in two components. First the function/symptom questions (30 items, scored 1–5) and second the optional high performance sports/work/musicians section (4 items, scored 1–5).

Function/Symptoms Score

The response to the first 30 items of the DASH are summed to form a raw score. The maximum score possible is 150, the minimum score is 30 (range of scores = 120). The raw score is 10 transformed to a 0 to 100 scale with 0 reflecting no disability (good function) and 100 reflecting a lot of disability.

To transform the score follow this formula:

Function/Sympton scale (30 items):

$$\frac{\text{Raw score} - 30 \text{ (minimum score)}}{1.20 \text{ (score range/100)}} = \text{DASH function/symptom score}$$

Appendix 1 (cont.)

Optional module

The optional module is made up of four items that may or may not be used by individuals because of the nature of the questions. The goal was to include the items in the DASH that would capture the very fine difficulties that professional musicians or athletes or workers might encounter in their occupation but that might not affect their activities of daily living.

The maximum score of this section is 20 with a minimum of 4. The range of scores is therefore 16. This score is also transformed to a 0 to 100 scale, with lower scores reflecting minimal disability and higher scores reflecting more disability.

Sports/Music/Work Optional Module (4 items):

$$\frac{\text{Raw score} - 4 \text{ (minimum score)}}{.16 \text{ (score range/100)}} = \textbf{DASH optional component score}$$

Missing items

If fewer than 10 percent of items (3 function/symptom questions) are left blank by the respondent, the mean (average) of the scores to the other items may be substituted in for this item. For instance, if a person responds with 28 "3" scores and two blanks, the missing values can be replaced by the value "3" as the mean of the other responses. If more than 10 percent are left blank, you will not be able to calculate a DASH score. By this same rule, no missing values can be tolerated in the high performance sport/work/music module (only 4 items).

Appendix 2
Shoulder Arthroplasty Home Instructions, Rehabilitation Services

GENERAL INSTRUCTIONS (4–6 WEEKS)

- The exercise program should be done _____ times a day.
- Increase the number of repetitions to 10.
- Do each exercise slowly and smoothly. You should feel a gentle stretch in each direction. It may be uncomfortable, but it should not be painful.
- Wear your arm sling at night until discontinued by your surgeon. Do not sleep on your operated arm.
- As an extra precaution, wear the sling out in public.
- Avoid reaching or lifting an object with your arm out to the side.
- Avoid pushing down with your operated arm when getting up from a chair, the toilet, or the bathtub.
- Use extra caution in the bathroom, and use equipment as instructed by your practitioner.
- When dressing, put the garment over your operated arm first and then onto the other arm. When undressing, remove the garment from the operated arm last.
- You may return to work and drive at the discretion of your surgeon.

Additional Instructions:

_____

_____

_____

Your surgeon will progress your exercise program at each postoperative visit. Be prepared with your questions. Write them down. Ask about lifting, sports, and other tasks important to you.

EXERCISES:

1. Hand, wrist, and elbow ROM
2. Pendulum movements
3. Shoulder internal rotation and external rotation in adduction
4. Supine active and assisted flexion
5. Supine assisted abduction
6. Sitting/standing: hand to mouth, hand to nose, hand to forehead _____ times
7. Program may include one or more of the following depending on surgical precautions:
   - isometrics
   - Shoulder pulleys
   - Unlimited active movement

Note. From Brigham and Women's Hospital, Boston, MA. Reprinted with permission.

Appendix 3
Sample of a Progressive Exercise Program for a Shoulder Arthroplasty

GROUP INTO THE FOLLOWING SECTIONS:

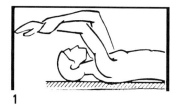

1

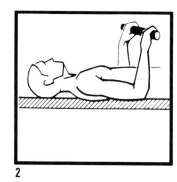

2

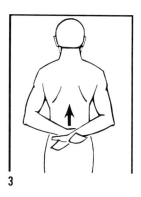

3

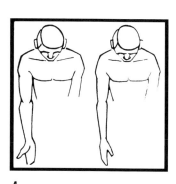

4

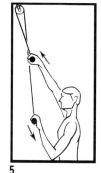

5

Assisted motions (A)
1. Flexion: supine
2. External rotation: supine (moving dowel side to side)
3. Internal rotation in extension: standing
4. Pendulum and combined motions: leaning forward in sitting or standing supported
5. Elevation: standing or sitting with pulleys

Active motions (B)
1. Flexion: supine
2. Flexion: sitting
3. Elevation: standing and sitting

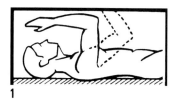

1

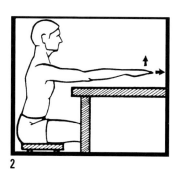

2

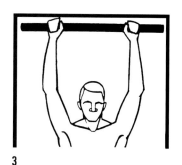

3

Appendix 3 (cont.)

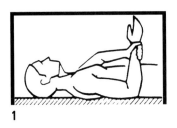

1

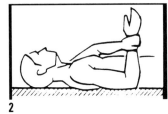

2

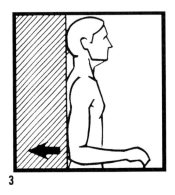

3

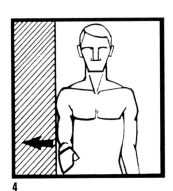

4

Strengthening—Isometrics (C)
1. Internal rotation: supine, progress to sitting and standing
2. External rotation: supine, progress to sitting and standing
3. Extension: standing and sitting
4. Abduction: standing

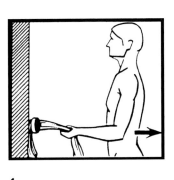

1

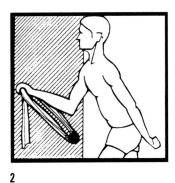

2

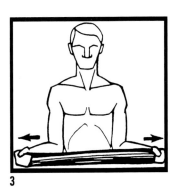

3

Strengthening—With Theraband™ (D)
(These will have to be adapted for PTs with hand and elbow involvement)
1. Extension: standing
2. Flexion and elevation: standing (This is difficult and is not advised if the rotator cuff is not intact or functioning well.)
3. External rotation and scapula retraction: supine or standing

Note. Sketches used with permission of Biomet, Inc., Warsaw, IN.

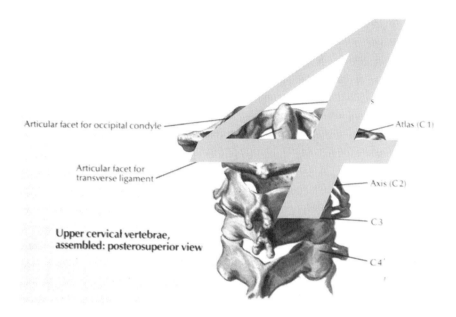

Articular facet for occipital condyle

Atlas (C 1)

Articular facet for
transverse ligament

Axis (C 2)

C 3

**Upper cervical vertebrae,
assembled: posterosuperior view**

C 4

RHEUMATOID ARTHRITIS OF THE SPINE:
SURGERY AND REHABILITATION

James Coyle, MD, Rick B. Delamarter, MD, and Jeanne L. Melvin, MS, OTR, FAOTA

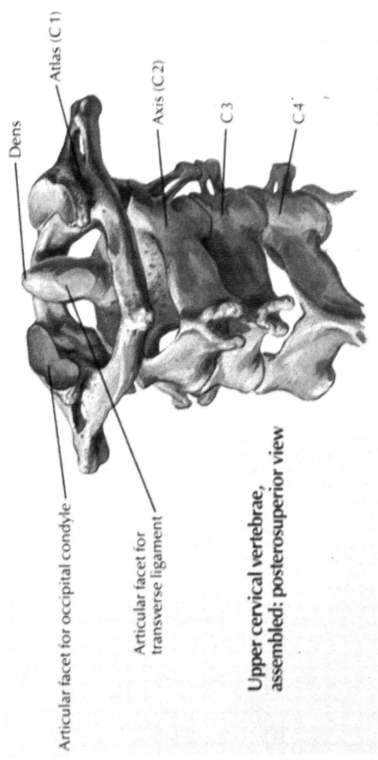

Dens

Atlas (C1)

Axis (C2)

C 3

C 4

Articular facet for occipital condyle

Articular facet for transverse ligament

Upper cervical vertebrae, assembled: posterosuperior view

Anatomy of the upper cervical vertebrae—posterosuperior view. Copyright 1989. Novartis. Reprinted with permission from the *Atlas of Human Anatomy*, illustrated by Frank H. Netter, MD. All rights reserved.

The manifestations of rheumatoid arthritis (RA) in the spine are confined primarily to the cervical spine, with the principal area of involvement encompassing the occipitoatlantoaxial region or upper cervical spine. Articulations of the cervical spine are second only to metatarsophalangeal joints in frequency of involvement with RA (Agarwal, Peppelman, Kraus, Pollock, Stolzer, Eisenbeis, & Donaldson, 1992). Although cervical spine instability has been shown to be present in 43 to 86% of patients with RA (Boden, 1994), many of these patients are asymptomatic. When intractable pain and neurological compromise occur in the cervical spine as a result of arthritic changes, treatment can be one of the most challenging tasks in the care of the patient with RA. The consequences of instability and spinal cord compression may include severe myelopathy, progressive quadriparesis, and sudden death because of compression of the spinal cord or the cardiorespiratory centers in the brain stem.

The pathophysiology of RA as it affects the cervical spine is identical to the process affecting peripheral joints. Synovial inflammation leads to the formation of a pannus of granulation tissue and destruction of cartilage and ligamentous attachments. Along with erosion of bone, this results in destabilization of the cervical spine articulations, which causes instability, subluxation, and neurological dysfunction. In addition, the rheumatoid cervical spine may be severely osteoporotic, have erosive diskitis, and undergo spontaneous fusion between levels.

Anatomy

An appreciation of cervical spine anatomy is essential to understand how the progression of RA results in instability, subluxation, and neurological compromise. The first cervical vertebra is the atlas, or C1. It consists of two lateral masses connected by an anterior and a posterior arch. There is no vertebral body and no spinous process. It has been referred to as an *ossified meniscus* between the occiput and the axis, or C2. The superior facets are concave and articulate with the occipital condyles. The atlantoaxial articulation is responsible for about 50% of total cervical spine range of motion (ROM).

Within each lateral mass is a transverse foramen through which the vertebral artery courses. After exiting the C1 transverse foramen, the arteries continue along the posterior arch of C1 and then ascend into the foramen magnum. Below C1, each vertebral artery courses through transverse foramina in the lateral masses of C2 to C6. As a consequence, subluxation of the cervical spine can potentially disrupt the vertebral-basilar blood supply to the brain.

The axis is distinguished by the odontoid process that is embryologically the body of C1. The odontoid, or dens, is the pivot around which the atlas rotates. The atlantoaxial joint provides about 50% of total cervical spine rotation. The ligamentous complex connecting C1 and C2 provides support and stability while allowing maximum movement. The transverse ligament is the most important for stability. It passes posterior to the odontoid and attaches to the inner sides of the lateral masses of C1. Deep to this are the alar ligaments that stretch from the odontoid to the occipital condyles. They act to limit rotation and provide additional stability in flexion and extension. Important joints within the atlantoaxial complex are synovial joints anterior and posterior to the odontoid and bilateral facet joints between C1 and C2. When they become involved with RA, these joints undergo proliferation of inflammatory synovitis and formation of pannus. The disk spaces between each vertebral body in the cervical spine, along with joints of Luschka, provide the site of articulation between the vertebral bodies anteriorly.

The 3rd to 6th cervical vertebrae are similar in appearance and articulation. In addition to their anterior disk articulations, they articulate at the facet joints bilaterally and are stabilized by the posterior longitudinal ligament along the posterior aspects of the vertebral bodies and by the interspinous ligaments connecting the spinous processes at each level. Each motion segment contributes approximately 10% of total flexion, extension, and rotation to the entire cervical spine.

Clinical Manifestations

Rheumatoid involvement of the cervical spine is more frequently seen in patients with seropositive disease and rheumatoid nodules, longstanding disease, and severe peripheral disease. Patients usually have peripheral involvement of RA for at least 5 years before demonstrating symptoms of cervical spine involvement (Sculco, 1992). Furthermore, many patients will be symptomatic for many years with neck pain but without clinically significant instability. Neck pain is reported in 40 to 88% of persons with RA, and cervical subluxation has been observed in 43 to 86%, but neurological deficit is reported in only 7 to 34% (Boden, 1994). In a large series of patients surgically treated for cervical spine deformities, the average duration of RA was 19 years before the onset of atlantoaxial subluxation and subaxial subluxation and 22 years before the onset of superior migration of the odontoid (Peppelman, Kraus, Donaldson, & Agarwal, 1993). As with peripheral involvement, the symptoms of RA in the cervical spine, although generally progressive, are marked by periods of exacerbation and remission.

As mentioned, patients presenting with cervical spine involvement are often among the most severely afflicted patients with RA who have debilitating peripheral disease. At the same time, patients with notable neurological compromise because of deformity of the cervical spine may present with only mild subjective complaints. Neurological examination of these patients is difficult because it is not always possible to distinguish between neurological deficits and problems caused by multiple joint involvement. Patients may have inflamed peripheral joints, contractures, tendon ruptures, muscle wasting, or multiple arthroplasties or fusions. In these cases, it is difficult to evaluate long-tract signs such as hyperreflexia, loss of motor function, and, in some cases, focal sensory deficits. When loss of function and weakness are associated with joint disease, they can mask the insidious onset of cervical instability and neurological compromise, thus leading to a delay in diagnosis and treatment (Delamarter, Bolesta, & Bohlman, 1991). Studies by Delamarter and Bohlman (1994) of postmortem findings on patients with paralysis secondary to RA of the cervical spine found spinal cord compression to be the main cause of death in 10 of 11 patients. This suggests that once spinal and spinal cord compression occurs, if left untreated, the natural history is grave, and the frequency of sudden death as a result of spinal cord compression may be underestimated. If a

Table 1. Clinical Signs and Symptoms of C1 to C2 Subluxation

Pain and tenderness in the upper cervical spine with radiation of pain to the occipital area or forehead and eye area
Hyperreflexia in upper and lower extremities
Peripheral muscle atrophy
Focal sensory deficits
L'Hermitte's sign (i.e., shocks of electricity during cervical flexion)
Compression of vertebral arteries
Feeling of heaviness in the legs
Disturbance in fine motor function (recent onset)
Ataxia (recent decline in ambulation)
Bowel or bladder dysfunction

neurological deficit is suspected, signs and symptoms found on physical examination should not simply be attributed to peripheral disease. The physical exam should be followed by a radiographic evaluation to diagnose any evidence of cervical instability and spinal cord compression.

Cervical Subluxation

There are three main patterns of cervical subluxation resulting from RA:

1. atlantoaxial or C1 to C2 instability

2. basilar invagination

3. subaxial or rotatory subluxation

Atlantoaxial Subluxation

Atlantoaxial or C1 to C2 subluxation is the most common type of instability, involves 50 to 70% of cases (Table 1; Boden, Dodge, Bohlman, & Rechtine, 1993), and is usually anterior. Lateral subluxation occurs less commonly, and, in rare instances, with complete erosion or fracture of the odontoid, posterior subluxation can occur.

Atlantoaxial subluxation is primarily a result of an erosive synovitis of the C1 to C2 articulations, with pannus formation around the odontoid, and causes laxity or disruption of the transverse and alar ligaments. This allows forward displacement of the atlas on the axis, thus compressing the spinal cord between the odontoid and the posterior arch of C1. In the average cervical spine, the inner diameter of the ring of C1 is approximately 30 mm anterior to posterior, with 10 mm of space occupied by the odontoid and about 10 mm occupied by the spinal cord. In addition to the decrease in space that results from anterior subluxation, synovial pannus formation around the odontoid further reduces the space available for the spinal cord. With instability and compression of the spinal cord, irreversible neurological compromise may result. Although as many as 25% of hospitalized patients with RA may have radiographic evidence of atlantoaxial subluxation, the number of patients who develop neurological symptoms is much less, in the range of 2% to 14% (Simpson & Booth, 1992; Figure 1).

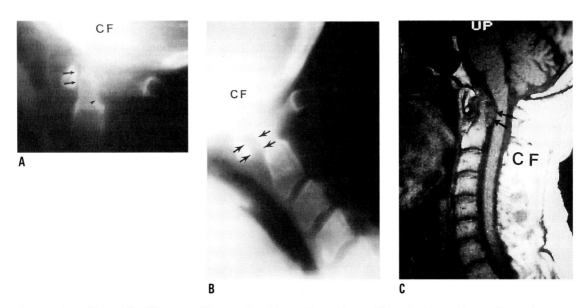

Figure 1. C1 to C2 instability. This woman (55 years of age) had a 15-year history of RA and a 10-year history of increasing neck pain. (A): Lateral radiograph of the C1 to C2 interval in extension. Note the odontoid is in its proper anatomic location up against the anterior arch of C1 (long arrows). Additionally note the erosion of the posterior aspect of the odontoid from the rheumatoid pannus (small arrows). (B): Flexion lateral radiograph. Note the subluxation of the odontoid behind the anterior arch of C1 (arrows). (C): MRI reveals major pannus surrounding the odontoid (lower arrow), which causes impingement of the upper cervical spinal cord (upper arrow). Major pannus around the odontoid can cause cervical spinal cord compression even without frank instability of the C1 to C2 segment.

Traditionally, when viewing a lateral cervical spine radiograph, the interval between the anterior arch of C1 and the odontoid, known as the anterior *atlanto-dens* or *atlanto-odontoid interval*, has been used to evaluate atlantoaxial instability. An atlanto-odontoid interval of greater than 3.5 mm is considered abnormal, and an interval greater than 10 mm implies disruption of the entire supporting ligamentous complex (Fielding, Cochran, Lawsing, & Hohl, 1974). Boden and colleagues (1993) have shown that the posterior atlanto-odontoid interval may provide a better correlation with the presence and severity of paralysis. The posterior atlanto-odontoid interval is measured between the posterior aspect of the odontoid and the posterior arch of C1 and represents the space available for the spinal cord.

Patients who present with symptomatic atlantoaxial instability may complain of headaches or neck and shoulder pain. Compression on the greater occipital nerves, which exit the spinal canal posteriorly between C1 and C2, will result in headaches primarily in the occipital region. Pain secondary to C1–C2 subluxation may radiate to the forehead and eyes (Delamarter et al., 1991). Patients may present with a sudden sensation of electricity radiating through the body and into the arms and legs, referred to as *L'Hermitte's sign*. This is elicited by cervical spine motion in flexion and extension. Signs of myelopathy as a result of cord compression include weakness and paresthesias in the extremities, a feeling of heaviness in the legs, new onset of difficulties with fine motor movements, stumbling or difficulties with gait, and bowel or bladder dysfunction. Patients presenting with such evidence of neurological compromise may be at risk for permanent paralysis and even sudden death. This situation requires prompt referral to a surgeon (Halla, 1997).

Ranawat, O'Leary, and Pellicci (1979) have provided a classification scheme for patients presenting with neurological deficits. Class I patients present with pain but no neurological deficit; Class II patients present with weakness, hyperreflexia, and dysesthesia; and Class III patients have paresis and long-tract findings and are further divided into two groups: Class IIIA patients are ambulatory, and Class IIIB patients are nonambulatory. In general, the more severe the rheumatologic deformity and instability, the more severe the neurological involvement is. Several studies have found Ranawat's classification scheme to be a useful prognostic tool in that patients with more severe deficits have less recovery and have higher perioperative morbidity and mortality rates. As a rule, neurological recovery in patients with myelopathy is poor (Peppelman et al., 1993; Santavirta et al., 1991).

On presentation, any patient suspected of having a neurological deficit should undergo urgent radiographic evaluation of the site of neurological compromise. Initial evaluation of instability is obtained with plain radiographs and includes an anteroposterior view, an open-mouth odontoid view, and lateral flexion and extension films. Magnetic resonance imaging (MRI) is the best modality for visualizing soft tissue and is useful for demonstrating synovial pannus formation and spinal cord and brain stem compression. The indications for surgery for atlantoaxial subluxation include intractable pain and neurological deficit. The use of radiographic evidence of instability as an indication for surgery has been more controversial. Although some authors recommend not undertaking prophylactic stabilization on the basis of radiographic instability in the absence of a neurological deficit, others have concluded that surgical stabilization should be considered in patients with severe instability before the onset of irreversible neurological changes (Peppelman et al., 1993). Boden (1994) has noted that, in patients without a neurological deficit, it is generally safe to continue observation if the posterior atlanto-odontoid interval measures greater than 14 mm on plain radiographs. If, however, the interval is less than 14 mm, an MRI is warranted. Furthermore, if the MRI shows a cord diameter less than 6 mm in flexion or a space available for the cord of less than 13 mm, a fusion should be considered.

Surgical stabilization is most commonly accomplished by posterior arthrodesis of C1 to C2. Several techniques have been described, the most common being the Gallie fusion or a variation of the Gallie fusion. In this operation, the posterior lamina of the atlas and axis are exposed, and 20-gauge wire is passed under the lamina of the atlas and secured over an autogenous iliac crest bone graft to the spinous process of the axis (see Figure 2).

It is frequently necessary to reduce the C1 to C2 subluxation before performing the arthrodesis. For this purpose, preoperative halo traction or placement of a halo vest may be necessary. In those instances in which subluxation is fixed and contributing to spinal cord compression, it may be necessary to decompress posteriorly by removing the posterior arch of the atlas and extending the fusion to the occiput. Postoperatively, patients are maintained in a halo vest until the fusion heals, a period from 3 to 4 months.

Fusion rates range from 60 to 100% and predictably achieve pain relief, but recovery from preoperative myelopathy is limited (Chan, Ngian, & Cohen, 1992). Santavirta and colleagues (1991) followed a group of patients who underwent Gallie fusions for 10 years. They noted that patients with long-term cortisone treatment were more likely to develop a pseudoarthrosis or nonunion of the fusion, but they found no correlation between clinical outcome and radiographic result.

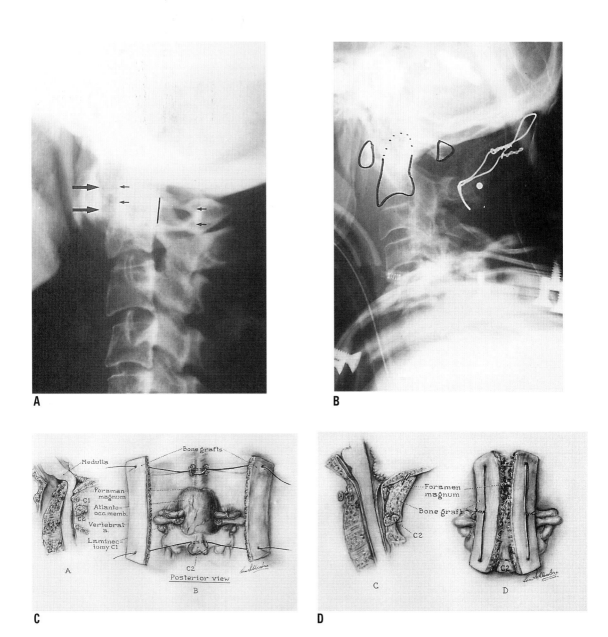

Figure 2. A woman (62 years of age) with a 14-year history of RA had a 5-year history of progressive neck pain and a 1-year history of progressive weakness of the arms and legs. (A): Lateral radiograph in the neutral position reveals a C1 to C2 instability with an anterior dens interval of approximately 8 mm (large arrows) and a space available for the cord of 13 mm instead of the normal 20 mm. Note the tip of the odontoid is not well visualized, which suggests basilar invagination. (B): Postoperative lateral radiograph reveals a typical occipital to C2 spinal fusion with wire fixation of iliac crest-bone graft between the occiput to the C2 vertebral body. (There are two separate wires [2D]). The patient is kept in a rigid cervical orthosis postoperatively for 2 to 3 months. The anterior and posterior arch of C1 and the odontoid are outlined. (C): Illustration of a occipital cervical fusion. Note the posterior arch of C1 has been removed and wires placed into the base of the occiput as well as through the C2 spinous process. (D): Completion of the fusion with wiring of the iliac crest strut grafts directly on the occiput to the C2 vertebra. Note the decompressed spinal cord. Excellent fusion rates can be expected with this technique.

Basilar Invagination

Basilar invagination is the least common but potentially the most devastating type of cervical instability resulting from rheumatoid involvement of the cervical spine. Basilar invagination is likewise referred to as *superior migration of the odontoid, cranial settling*, or *atlantoaxial impaction*. Basilar invagination is almost always seen in combination with atlantoaxial subluxation and occurs because of disruption of the ligamentous complex stabilizing the occipitoatlantoaxial joints along with bony and cartilaginous erosions. The lateral masses of the atlas may collapse and lead to vertical subluxation of the odontoid process through the foramen magnum. The odontoid process, which may be enveloped in synovial pannus, can compress the cervical medullary junction. Basilar invagination may affect as many as 10% of patients with RA in the cervical spine (see Figure 3).

Basilar invagination traditionally has been diagnosed with plain radiographs by using the lateral X ray. Several radiographic indexes have been described. For example, McGregor's line, which extends from the posterior margin of the hard pallet to the most caudal point of the occiput, can be used. A projection of the odontoid of more than 4.5 mm above McGregor's line is characteristic of basilar invagination. Other indexes of basilar invagination include McRae's line, Chamberlain's line, and the Ranawat index. All of these indexes are limited by the difficulty in visualizing the tip of the odontoid and landmarks in the base of the skull on plain X rays. The use of MRI to evaluate basilar invagination may provide more accurate imaging of both the extent of vertical subluxation of the odontoid and associated pannus and the extent of spinal cord and brain stem compression.

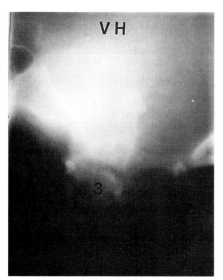
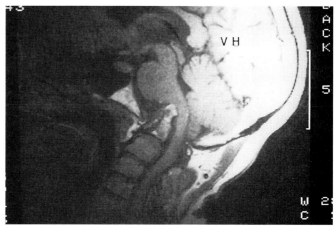

Figure 3. Basilar invagination for a woman (58 years of age) with a 20-year history of RA presented with a 3-year history of progressive neck pain and difficulty ambulating with weakness of the arms and legs. She has severe erosive disease in her hands, wrists, and feet. (A): Lateral tomogram of the occipital–cervical junction. Note the C3 vertebra is at the base of the occiput, and the entire odontoid is migrated into the foramen magnum, thus revealing severe basilar invagination. (B): MRI shows severe basilar invagination with migration of the odontoid into the foramen magnum with severe cervical medullary junction compression. The patient was treated with 1 week of halo traction and an occipital to C2 fusion with excellent neurological recovery.

Patients with basilar invagination may present with any or all of the neurological sequelae associated with atlantoaxial subluxation, including progressive myelopathy, vertebral artery thrombosis, and sudden death. In general, patients with basilar invagination have more severe neurological deficits, and there is less neurological recovery after stabilization. Peppelman and associates (1993) have noted that earlier C1 to C2 fusions for atlantoaxial subluxation may play a role in preventing the development of basilar invagination and neurological findings. They recommend performing fusion earlier, before the development of basilar invagination and neurological deficits.

Surgical stabilization of basilar invagination involves occiput-to-axis arthrodesis. Some surgeons use a preoperative period of halo traction to obtain reduction of the impaction and pull the odontoid from the foramen magnum (Delamarter et al., 1991). Others believe that atlantoaxial impaction is usually fixed and that attempting to reduce it with preoperative traction is not helpful (Sculco, 1992). However, in one large series, most Ranawat Class IIIB patients improved to Class IIIA or better before surgery with the application of a halo and reduction alone, which eliminated some of the cord compression (Peppelman et al., 1993). It has been shown that, with a solid fusion, there is a spontaneous reduction in the synovial pannus around the odontoid, as visualized on MRI (Moskovich, 1991). Occasionally, if there is compression of the spinal cord or brain stem posteriorly, it may be necessary to decompress the posterior arch of the atlas and the foramen magnum. For anterior decompression, resection of the odontoid by a transoral or retropharyngeal approach can be performed, but these procedures are associated with high morbidity and mortality rates and are rarely indicated (Morgan & Murphy, 1992).

Subaxial or Rotary Subluxation

Subaxial or rotary subluxation is typically a late development and can be defined as translation of one vertebral body in relation to an adjacent vertebral body below C2 (White, Johnson, Panhjabi, & Southwick, 1975). A more clinically relevant measurement may be the posterior subaxial canal diameter or the space available for the cord (Boden, 1994). Subaxial subluxation may affect multiple levels of vertebrae and lead to a step-ladder deformity (Simpson & Booth, 1992). Subaxial subluxation may be the result of synovitic destruction of facet joints, ligamentous laxity, and erosive diskitis. It is frequently seen in conjunction with atlantoaxial subluxation and basilar invagination in complex rheumatoid deformities of the cervical spine. It may follow spontaneous autofusions of adjacent levels as a result of increased stresses placed on the subluxing level. Kraus and associates have noted a 36% subaxial subluxation rate after a mean of 2.6 years in patients who have had fusion from the occiput to C3 for atlantoaxial subluxation and basilar invagination (Kraus, Peppelman, Agarwal, DeLeeuw, & Donaldson, 1991). Patients who present with combinations of atlantoaxial instability, basilar invagination, and subaxial subluxation should have the entire spectrum of their deformity addressed during the same surgery, including all abnormal segments.

Stirrat and Fyfe (1993) have highlighted the usefulness of the halo jacket in the perioperative treatment of subaxial instability. The halo jacket allows stabilization and reduction of displacement, and both anterior and posterior surgical procedures can be performed in the halo jacket if necessary.

The most common surgical procedure for subaxial subluxations is posterior fusion. Autogenous iliac crest bone graft is used, along with various techniques that use spinous process wiring or lateral mass plates. A laminectomy may be indicated in areas of posterior compression of the spinal cord;

anterior diskectomy and fusion as a second-stage procedure is rarely indicated (Delamarter, et al., 1991, p. 757). The indications for surgery are the same as those for upper surgical subluxation; likewise, the goals of surgery are to stabilize the spine, relieve pain, and prevent the onset of irreversible neurological deficits.

Planning for Surgery

Most patients who need cervical surgery have severe RA and are on multiple anti-inflammatory and immunosuppressive medications. Medication changes are coordinated with the treating rheumatologist. Generally, we prefer to stop nonsteroidal anti-inflammatory drugs (NSAIDs), which can potentiate bleeding, for several weeks before a fusion to limit blood loss during surgery; likewise, we avoid using NSAIDs for several months after surgery to reduce the risk of nonunion. Methotrexate has been associated with decreased wound healing. It is stopped 1 week before surgery and withheld for 1 to 2 weeks postoperatively. Corticosteroids are continued up to the preoperative day, and the patient is given a stress dose of intravenous hydrocortisone perioperatively.

Presurgical functional evaluation is helpful for planning postoperative rehabilitation. Patients with severe RA often compensate for loss of shoulder or elbow flexion by flexing their neck (e.g., to reach their mouth when feeding or to wash the top of their head). When this is the case, cervical fusion in neutral can be expected to reduce their functional ability. For the severely limited patient, preoperative self-care evaluation while wearing a collar or sitting in traction can determine if cervical fusion will impair functional ability. This allows for planning therapy to improve function either through exercise or assistive devices.

Preoperative evaluation must include a plan for having someone in the home help the patient with self-care and homemaking while the patient is in the halo cast. Patients with rheumatoid involvement of their shoulders and elbows may experience exacerbation of their symptoms or a decrease in function as a result of wearing the halo vest. This must be discussed with the patient before surgery so that he or she is aware of all the risks.

Preoperative evaluation of the patient's functional status is important because most patients will be required to wear a halo vest for 3 to 4 months after surgery. Family members or caregivers must be trained to pay careful attention to pin site care and areas of pressure on the skin once the halo vest is applied. Particular emphasis should be paid to ROM of the upper extremities.

Surgical Rehabilitation

The perioperative and postoperative periods for patients undergoing surgical stabilization of rheumatoid deformities of the cervical spine can be fraught with complications. Patients are particularly susceptible to pulmonary complications postoperatively, and in the case of patients taking chronic corticosteroids or immunosuppressants, an increased incidence of wound infections and sepsis is common. Great care must be exercised during operative positioning and induction of anesthesia to prevent these complications.

Early postoperative mobilization is essential to reduce the incidence of postsurgical complications. A rehabilitation plan that incorporates the expertise of the surgeon, nursing staff members, and occupational and physical therapy practitioners is essential for maximizing the rehabilitation potential of the patient postoperatively. Discharge planning should begin before or on the first day of admission. In a managed care environment, length of stay for an anterior cervical fusion is 2 to 5 days. Postoperative therapy includes gentle active ROM to the upper extremities, muscle strengthening, ambulation training, activities of daily living (ADL) evaluation, and training to maximize functional independence. Because most patients requiring cervical fusion have severe disabilities and are not independent in ADL, they are transferred to a subacute or full rehabilitation unit for 1 to 3 weeks. The focus of therapy in rehabilitation is on the previously discussed interventions and expands to include muscle reeducation, dexterity, and sensory reeducation.

Fortunately, the halo and vest traction devices are not needed in all cases. When they are used, patients need advice, equipment, and training in all areas of ADL. Acquiring a comfortable sleep position is often a major challenge. Some patients have found it helpful to place a Jackson Cervipillo™ (made by the Trueze Company) between their neck and the posterior two bars for support. Egg crate foam mattress pads can likewise increase comfort (Melvin, 1989).

Devices such as a reading rack can make reading a feasible and comfortable leisure activity. It is important to keep in mind that patients with fused necks have a restricted peripheral view, so they must turn their entire body to see to the side. This is not only an inefficient use of energy but also painful for patients with stiff joints or limited ROM. One of the most valuable home aids for these patients is a comfortable, safe chair with a swivel base. This provides an effortless rotation ability to participate in conversations and to view activities around the house. For example, a swivel chair in the living room allows these patients to see what is happening in the dining room or kitchen without having to stand up. Executive office chairs with the caster wheels removed work well for this purpose. If the patient returns to driving, a wide extension for the rear-view mirror and side mirrors must be installed to ensure adequate peripheral vision (Melvin, 1989).

Finally, patients who are ambulatory are at increased risk for falls during the period in which they use the halo vest. The risk can be minimized by emphasizing postoperative gait training and by using assistive devices, including the rolling walker and quad cane.

Thoracic and Lumbar Spine

The incidence of lower-back pain lasting longer than 3 months occurs with the same frequency in patients with RA as it does in the general population (Helliwell, Zaboani, Porter, & Wright, 1993). There is, however, a higher incidence of insufficiency fractures in patients with RA. Spector, Hall, McCloskey, and Karis (1993) found the rate of vertebral fractures in postmenopausal women with RA to be twice that in age-matched control subjects (12% vs. 6.5%).

Spinal Stenosis

Lumbar spinal stenosis is characterized by a decrease in the dimensions of the spinal canal and neural foramen. An extensive list of factors is implicated in the causes of spinal stenosis, including osteoarthritis, congenital developmental stenosis, postoperative stenosis, ankylosing spondylitis, and RA (Moreland, Lopez-Mendez, & Alarcon, 1989). Patients with spinal stenosis typically present with lower-back pain and pain radiating to the buttocks, thighs, calves, and feet. Symptoms are increased by ambulation and posture that decreases the diameter of the spinal canal. The symptom complex is referred to as *neurogenic claudication*. Patients typically gain relief of symptoms by forward flexion against a table or ambulating while leaning over a walker or shopping cart. The forward-flexed posture results in an increase in spinal canal diameter, thus relieving symptoms of claudication.

Spinal stenosis typically is diagnosed in patients between 50 and 70 years of age. Computed tomography myelography is the most useful modality for visualization of the bony architecture of spinal stenosis, whereas MRI provides excellent definition of soft-tissue structures, including disk herniations and ligamentum flavum thickening.

Nonoperative treatment of spinal stenosis is the initial approach and includes use of nonsteroidal medications, physical therapy, lumbar arthrosis, and epidural steroid injections. The relief provided by conservative measures, including epidural steroid injections, is usually transient, however, and definitive treatment requires surgical decompression. Several studies of surgical decompression demonstrate good to excellent results in 75% to 85% of cases (Delamarter & Howard, 1993).

Summary

RA of the cervical spine can result in major disability. Spinal instability with myleopathy left untreated can result in quadriparesis and sudden death. Practitioners treating patients for peripheral RA are in an unique position to screen patients for cervical instability and nerve compression and to refer the patient to his or her physician for further evaluation. Early referral for surgical stabilization optimizes functional outcome. Surgical fusion has been proven to be the only predictable intervention to stop the progression of cranial settling and cord compression in the cervical spine.

References

Agarwal, A. K., Peppelman, W. C., Kraus, D. R., Pollock, B. H., Stolzer, B. L., Eisenbeis, C. H. Jr., & Donaldson, W. F. III. (1992). Recurrence of cervical spine instability in rheumatoid arthritis following previous surgery: Can disease progression be prevented by early surgery? *Journal of Rheumatology, 19*(9), 1364–1370.

Boden, S. D. (1994). Rheumatoid arthritis of the cervical spine: Surgical decision making based on predictors of paralysis and recovery. *Spine, 19*(20), 2275–2280.

Boden, S. D., Dodge, L. D., Bohlman, H. H., & Rechtine, G. R. (1993). Rheumatoid arthritis of the cervical spine: A long-term analysis with predictors of paralysis and recovery. *Journal of Bone and Joint Surgery, 75A*, 1282–1297.

Chan, D. P. K., Ngian, K. S., & Cohen, L. (1992). Posterior upper cervical fusion in rheumatoid arthritis. *Spine, 17*(3), 268–272.

Delamarter, R. B., & Bohlman, H. H. (1994). Postmortem osseous and neuropathologic analysis of the rheumatoid cervical spine. *Spine, 19*(20), 2267–2274.

Delamarter, R. B., Bolesta, M. J., & Bohlman, H. H. (1991). Rheumatoid arthritis: Surgical treatment. In J. W. Frymoyer (Ed.), *The adult spine: Principles and practice* (pp. 745–762). New York: Raven Press.

Delamarter, R. B., & Howard, M. W. (1993). Lumbar spinal stenosis. In S. H. Hochschuler & H. B. Cotler (Eds.), *Rehabilitation of the spine: Science and practice* (pp. 443–456). St. Louis, MO: Mosby.

Fielding, J. W., Cochran, G. van B., Lawsing, J. F. III, & Hohl, M. (1974). Tears of the transverse ligament of the atlas: A clinical and biomechanical study. *Journal of Bone and Joint Surgery, 56A,* 1683–1691.

Halla, J. (1997). Rheumatologic emergencies. *Bulletin on the Rheumatic Diseases, 46*(1), 4–6.

Helliwell, P. S., Zeboani, L. N. P., Porter, G., & Wright, V. (1993). A clinical and radiological study of back pain in rheumatoid arthritis. *British Journal of Rheumatology, 32,* 216–221.

Kraus, D. R., Peppelman, W. C., Agarwal, A. K., DeLeeuw, H. W., & Donaldson, W. F. III. (1991). Incidence of subaxial subluxation in patients with generalized rheumatoid arthritis who have had previous occipital cervical fusions. *Spine, 16* (Suppl.), 5486–5489.

Melvin, J. L. (1989). *Rheumatic disease in the adult and child: Occupational therapy and rehabilitation* (3rd ed.). Philadelphia: F. A. Davis.

Moreland, L. W., Lopez-Mendez, A., & Alarcon, G. S. (1989). Spinal stenosis: A comprehensive review of the literature. *Seminars in Arthritis and Rheumatism, 19*(2), 127–149.

Morgan, S., & Murphy, G. (1992). The transoral approach to the cervical spine. *Journal of Neuroscience Nursing, 24*(5), 269–272.

Moskovich, R. (1991). Cervical instability. In K. H. Bridwell, R. L. Dewald, & K. W. Hammerberg (Eds.), *Textbook of spine surgery* (p. 819). Philadelphia: Lippincott.

Peppelman, W. C., Kraus, D. R., Donaldson, W. F. III, & Agarwal, A. (1993). Cervical spine surgery in rheumatoid arthritis: Improvement of neurologic deficit after cervical spine fusion. *Spine, 18*(16), 2375–2379.

Ranawat, C. S., O'Leary, P., & Pellicci, P. (1979). Cervical fusion in rheumatoid arthritis. *Journal of Bone and Joint Surgery, 61A,* 1003–1010.

Santavirta, S., Konttinen, Y. T., Laasonen, E., Honkanen, V., Antti-Poika, I., & Kauppi, M. (1991). Ten-year results of operations for rheumatoid cervical spine disorders. *Journal of Bone and Joint Surgery, 73B,* 116–120.

Sculco, T. (1992). *Surgical treatment of rheumatoid arthritis.* St Louis, MO: Mosby-Year Book.

Simpson, J. M., & Booth, R. (1992). Arthritis of the spine. In R. H. Rothman & F. A. Simeone, (Eds.), *The spine* (Vol. 1, 3rd ed., pp. 536–538). Philadelphia: Saunders.

Spector, T. D., Hall, G. M., McCloskey, E. V., & Karis, J. A. (1993). Risk of vertebral fracture in women with rheumatoid arthritis. *British Medical Journal, 306*(6877), 588.

Stirrat, A. N., & Fyfe, I. S. (1993). Surgery of the rheumatoid cervical spine: Correlation of the pathology and prognosis. *Clinical Orthopaedics and Related Research, 293,* 135–143.

White, A. A., Johnson, R. M., Panhjabi, M. M., & Southwick, W. O. (1975). Biomechanical analysis of clinical instability in the cervical spine. *Clinical Orthopaedics and Related Research, 109,* 85–96.

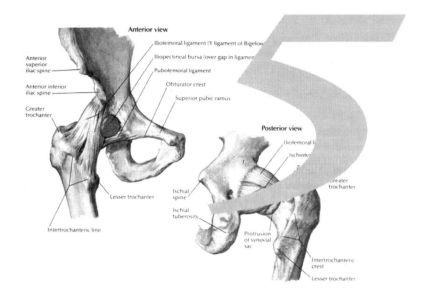

HIP SURGERY AND REHABILITATION

Scott David Martin, MD, Kathleen Zavadak, PT, Jill Noaker, OTR, CHT,
Mary Ann Jacobs, RN, and Robert Poss, MD

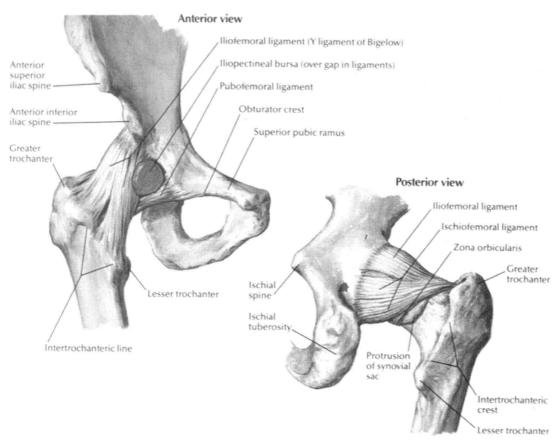

Anterior view

Iliofemoral ligament (Y ligament of Bigelow)

Iliopectineal bursa (over gap in ligaments)

Pubofemoral ligament

Obturator crest

Superior pubic ramus

Anterior superior iliac spine

Anterior inferior iliac spine

Greater trochanter

Lesser trochanter

Intertrochanteric line

Posterior view

Iliofemoral ligament

Ischiofemoral ligament

Zona orbicularis

Greater trochanter

Ischial spine

Ischial tuberosity

Protrusion of synovial sac

Intertrochanteric crest

Lesser trochanter

Anatomy of the hip—anterior and posterior views. Copyright 1989. Novartis. Reprinted with permission from the *Atlas of Human Anatomy*, illustrated by Frank H. Netter, MD. All rights reserved.

reatment options for the diseased hip are varied and range from medical and rehabilitative therapy with the goal of maintaining hip motion, strength, and function to total hip replacement, which reliably relieves pain, improves motion, and restores function. The American College of Rheumatology's "Guidelines for the Medical Management of Osteoarthritis of the Hip" are outlined in Table 1 (Hochberg et al., 1995). Patients with progressive hip pain that interferes with activities of daily living (ADL) despite proper medication and therapy usually are considered candidates for hip surgery. Decision making in surgical treatment depends on the underlying pathology and amount of joint destruction, patient age, expectations, and functional disability.

This chapter reviews the arthritides that are frequently treated with hip surgery, such as post traumatic arthritis, osteoarthritis (OA), rheumatoid arthritis (RA), osteonecrosis, and septic arthritis. Ankylosing spondylitis and psoriatic arthritis may additionally affect the hip, but surgery is not as common in these cases, and surgery and rehabilitation would be the same as for RA. The preferred surgical options for treating arthritis of the hip—osteotomy, arthroscopy, and total hip arthroplasty (THA)—are discussed, along with postoperative rehabilitation. Salvage procedures such as hip arthrodesis and resection arthroplasty are included, but the major rehabilitative focus is on THA because it is the most common hip surgery, with more than 200,000 performed annually in the United States.

Table 1. American College of Rheumatology Guidelines for Medical Management of Patients With Osteoarthritis of the Hip

Nonpharmacological therapy
Patient education
Self-management programs (e.g., arthritis self-help course)
Health professionals' social support via telephone contact
Weight loss (if overweight)
Physical therapy
ROM exercises
Strengthening exercises
Assistive devices for ambulation
Occupational therapy
Joint protection and energy conservation
Assistive devices for ADL
Aerobic aquatic exercise programs
Pharmacological therapy
Nonopioid analgesics (e.g., acetaminophen)
Nonsteroidal anti-inflammatory drugs
Opioid analgesics

Note. From "Guidelines for the medical management of osteoarthritis. Part 1: Osteoarthritis of the hip," by M. C. Hochberg, R. D. Altman, K. D. Brandt, B. M. Clark, P. A. Dieppe, M. R. Griffin, R. W. Moskowitz, and T. J. Schnitzer, 1995, *Arthritis & Rheumatism,* 38, pp. 1535–1540. Copyright 1995 by Lippincott-Raven Publishers. Reprinted with permission.

Anatomy and Biomechanics of the Hip Joint

The human hip is a ball-and-socket type joint in which the hemispherical femoral head fits into a concave acetabulum or socket. The acetabulum consists of bony and fibrous structures that give inherent stability to the hip joint, which is important in maintaining an erect posture. The joint is lubricated by synovial fluid that decreases the coefficient of friction and allows for efficient hip movement. The narrow femoral neck allows for a wide range of movements while preventing impingement of the femur against the acetabular rim. The overall shape of the hip joint varies throughout life, but in the undiseased hip, the joint remains congruent, which prevents abnormal load bearing (Gruebel-Lee, 1983).

The estimated joint contact force in the hip during single-leg stance ranges from 2–6 times body weight (Rohrle, Scholten, & Sigolotto, 1984; Williams & Svennsson, 1968). During the terminal stance phase of gait, the peak joint forces range from 4.1–6.9 times body weight (Brand, Crowninshield, & Wittstock, 1982; Rohrle et al., 1984). These weight-bearing forces are believed to be the primary stress factors that exacerbate hip joint disease and lead to attrition of the articular cartilage (Sledge, 1979). In addition, when the congruity of the hip is altered, abnormal stress on the joint cartilage leads to underlying bone thickening before the joint surfaces begin to deteriorate. Changes in blood flow at various stages of development, deterioration of the femoral head, and occurrence of disease make the hip joint vulnerable to pathological changes throughout life.

During surgical reconstruction of the hip, the anatomy is altered to a certain extent with the goal of achieving maximal efficiency of the joint and the muscles acting across the hip. These alterations in anatomy sometimes involve changes in the muscle-moment arm, which subsequently changes the muscle tension and hip joint contact pressures. The magnitude of the moment that can be generated by a muscle is equal to the force produced by the muscle multiplied by the moment arm. The moment arm is defined as the perpendicular distance from the line of action of the muscle force to the axis of rotation, which is the center of the hip joint (Wickiewicz, Roy, Powell, & Edgerton, 1983).

Radiographic Examination

Radiographic analysis of the hip joint consists of an anteroposterior radiograph of the pelvis including both hips. This allows evaluation of the lesser trochanteric region of both hips and allows templating of the normal or less-involved hip to ensure proper sizing of the components and appropriate leg length. Templating is part of preoperative planning for all procedures. Besides determining the size of the implant, it will determine the orientation of the osteotomy cuts and placement of the fixation hardware. Templating will additionally determine the need for custom implants for smaller bones or bones with defects (Brower, 1994).

Lumbosacral spine and or ipsilateral knee radiographs should be obtained if those structures are believed to contribute to the patient's pain. If, after review of the radiographs, the contribution of hip pain from arthritis is still questionable, the patient should undergo a hip aspiration arthrogram with injection of an anesthetic to evaluate diagnostic relief and therapeutic benefit.

Disease Manifestations

The hip joint consists of the articular hyaline cartilage that coats the ends of all bones and a synovial lining. Joints comprise a mechanical system of ligaments, tendons, and muscles that together provide for proper functioning of the joint. Once cartilage injury occurs, repair takes place by either cloning of chondrocytes within the damaged cartilage or by proliferation of new cartilage from the underlying bone or the periphery of the joint. Proliferating new cartilage is usually more cellular, and matrix constituents may differ chemically and organizationally from normal articular cartilage. Over time, these differences can have an adverse effect on the function of the cartilage and may lead to the degradation of the joint surfaces (Sledge, 1979; Tsahakis, Brick, & Poss, 1993).

Posttraumatic arthritis may result from physical injury such as a fracture that extends into the joint surfaces. If an osteochondral injury occurs, a cartilage fragment (loose body) may injure the articular surface, which results in deterioration of the joint. Normal articular cartilage is highly resilient and can withstand cyclic loading without injury (Radin, Ehrlich, & Chernack, 1978; Repo & Finley, 1977). Despite this resilience, there is believed to be a threshold deformity that results in chondrocyte death (Repo & Finley, 1977). If the initial energy absorbed by the cartilage exceeds this critical threshold, chondrocyte death may occur and lead to traumatic arthritis (Upadhay & Moulton, 1981; Upadhay, Moulton, & Srikrishnamurthy, 1983). In addition, any major loss of normal articular congruence or articular contact secondary to defects or irregularities of the joint may predispose the joint to the development of early degenerative arthritis (Radin et al., 1978; Repo & Finley, 1977).

Fracture of the femoral head or acetabulum usually occurs after high-energy trauma. The goals of initial treatment include restoration of normal anatomy with perfect reduction of the joint surfaces if displacement has occurred. Even when these goals are achieved, acetabular and femoral head fractures may result in a rate of posttraumatic degenerative changes ranging as high as 57% of fractures in some reports (e.g., Carnesale, Stewart, & Barnes, 1975; Pennal, Davidson, Garside, & Plewes, 1980; Rowe & Lowell, 1961). In addition, avascular necrosis of the femoral head may occur in 2% to 40% and results in severe degenerative changes of the hip joint (Lachiewicz & Desman, 1988; Stewart & Milford, 1954; Urist, 1948).

Osteonecrosis, sometimes referred to as *avascular necrosis*, is a frequent cause of degenerative hip joint disease in younger patients (Figure 1A). It occurs more frequently in men than women, and, although there is a wide age distribution, most patients are less than 50 years of age (Calandriello & Grassi, 1982). Osteonecrosis is a condition in which there is a circulatory impairment of an area of bone that leads to its eventual death. There are many theories regarding etiology, most of which are formulated on the premise that an interruption of the normal blood supply to bone cells occurs (Fisher, 1978; Fisher & Bickel, 1971; Warner, Philip, Brodsky, & Thornhill, 1987).

Osteonecrosis can additionally be associated with systemic conditions that tend to produce unhealthy bone cells. Examples of systemic diseases that may lead to cell stress are systemic lupus erythematosus, asthma, chronic renal failure, and sickle cell disease. In 20% of patients, the cause of osteonecrosis is idiopathic, with no causal link. In nontraumatic cases, the incidence of bilateral disease is 50% to 80%. There are many other factors that may be associated with osteonecrosis, including

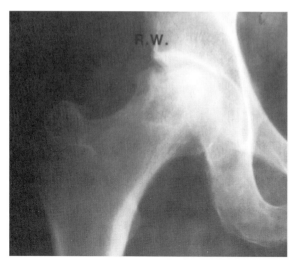

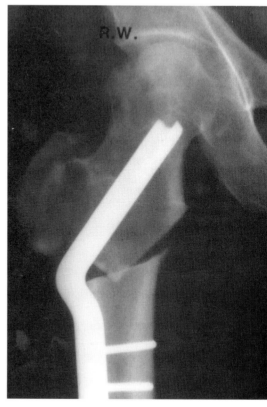

Figure 1. (A, above): Preoperative anteroposterior radiograph of idiopathic osteonecrosis of the femoral head in a man 33 years of age. (B, right): Postoperative anteroposterior radiograph of same patient treated with intertrochanteric osteotomy.

steroid use, alcohol use, and smoking. A thorough review is beyond the scope of this chapter but can be found in rheumatology and orthopedic texts (Marvin, 1993; Mazieres, 1994).

Early treatment of osteonecrosis is controversial and includes drilling or core decompression, decompression and bone grafting with either cortical or cancellous graft, and decompression and grafting with a free vascularized fibular graft. When collapse of the subchondral bone of the affected area occurs, treatment is limited to rotational osteotomy where the femur is osteotomized and healthier cartilage is rotated into the weight-bearing area (Figure 1B) (Sugioka & Ogata, 1991; Sugioka, Hotokebuchi, & Hideki, 1992). Other options include THA and, if that is not possible, arthrodesis. The literature currently supports THA versus hemiarthroplasty of the hip for late stages of osteonecrosis when disability and pain cannot be managed satisfactorily with conservative treatment (Figure 2) (Klaue, Durnin, & Ganz, 1991).

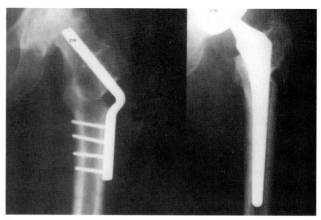

Figure 2. Anteroposterior radiographs of failed intertrochanteric osteotomy (*left*) converted to uncemented total hip arthroplasty (*right*).

Septic arthritis results from a bacterial infection of the joint. The acute inflammatory infiltrate from a bacterial joint infection produces proteolytic enzymes that can break down articular cartilage rapidly. Usually the patient will present with great pain and variable amounts of swelling of the joint. On clinical examination, the pain may be out of proportion to clinical findings with severe pain on attempted movement (Goldenberg, 1993). Frequently, with septic arthritis of the hip joint, the patient may find hip flexion with slight external rotation to be more comfortable because this position relaxes the joint capsule, thus decreasing the intra-articular pressure. Constitutional symptoms indicating septicemia (e.g., fever, chills, night sweats, malaise) are common. Joint aspiration reveals a predominance of polymorphonuclear leukocytes with a white blood cell count of more than 100,000. The most common bacteria to cause a joint infection is *Staphylococcus*; however, any bacteria has the potential to cause a joint infection. Treatment consists of antibiotic drugs, urgent open debridement, and lavage of the hip joint. If there is no septicemia, arthroscopy may be used instead of open surgery. Antibiotics are continued for 6 weeks.

OA is recognized as the most common joint disorder in humans. It is a process of gradual attrition of the articular cartilage surfaces of joints and growth of bone around the margins of the joint. The degeneration process leads to gradual loss of cartilage, which results in joint space narrowing on radiographs. The process is actually more complicated than simply a wearing away of cartilage but includes the reaction of the joint tissues to injury (Figure 3). The histological changes result from cell injury and the reparative or reactive changes that accompany the injury. Even though there are many types of arthritis, similar histological responses may be seen in the affected joint, regardless of the etiology (Brandt & Mankin, 1993; Gruebel-Lee, 1983).

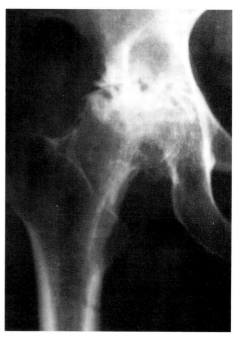

Figure 3. Anteroposterior radiograph demonstrating severe OA of right hip. Note large cyst formation in acetabulum with flattened femoral head and osteophyte formation.

RA is an inflammatory arthritis mainly of the peripheral joints that can result in major joint destruction and deformity. The hip is affected in 50% of patients (Brower, 1994). Unlike noninflammatory arthritis, with RA there is little reparative activity; therefore, osteophytes and new bone formation are not prominent but may occur as part of coexistent OA. Patients develop a hypertrophied and inflamed synovium, which may extend over the articular surface (pannus) and destroy the underlying cartilage by enzymatic degradation of the matrix. The rheumatoid synovium may invade and destroy the joint capsule and other periarticular supportive tissue, which results in marked instability with subluxation or dislocation of the involved joint (Poss & Sledge, 1981). In severe cases, the femur and acetabulum may migrate or protrude into the pelvis, referred to as *protrusio acetabuli*, and this occurs in 15% of patients with RA (Brower, 1994). In the late or end stages of RA, the affected joint may present with major destruction but with little inflammation or swelling and may be indistinguishable from OA.

Surgical Options

Osteotomy

An intertrochanteric osteotomy is performed in patients with hip dysplasia who have a deformed proximal femur and in isolated cases of idiopathic OA of the hip (Figure 4A). The osteotomy is carried out between the greater and lesser trochanteric regions to maximize proximal correction of the deformity and to provide a broad cancellous surface to encourage bony union (Figure 4B). The osteotomy allows the surgeon to move an area of the femoral head with remaining cartilage under the weight-bearing region of the hip. Fixation of the osteotomy site is carried out with a blade plate, which is used to assist in accurately correcting the proximal femur as templated during preoperative planning. Examination of the hip under fluoroscopy is advised to determine the proper surgical correction required to improve the radiographic joint space.

A recent retrospective review of 5 to 10-year follow-up of intertrochanteric osteotomies revealed improved results in hips with minimal preoperative radiographic change of osteoarthrosis. In addition, in hips with congenital dysplasia, the best results were in hips with the least degree of acetabular dysplasia (Perleau, Wilson, & Poss, 1996).

Periacetabular osteotomy is a procedure involving reorientation of the bone around the acetabulum. It allows multidirectional rotational correction of the acetabulum to improve coverage of the femoral head. In addition, the procedure allows medial displacement of the hip center, which decreases the hip joint reaction forces. When a concomitant valgus deformity of the femoral neck shaft angle exists, an adjuvant varus or varus extension osteotomy of the femur may be performed (Figures 4A and 4B) to correct architectural abnormalities of the acetabulum that are associated with minimal or no radiographic evidence of secondary arthritis (Sugioka et al., 1992; Trousdale, Ekkernkamp, & Ganz, 1995).

The most common indication for periacetabular osteotomy is a young patient with congenital dysplasia of the hip in which the acetabulum, femur, or both develop abnormally (Figure 4A). In these cases, symptoms may be related to labral tears of the acetabulum. However, repair of the labral tear does not correct the underlying problem of dysplasia (Klaue, Durnin, & Ganz, 1991). In con-

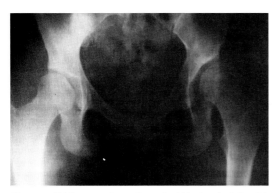 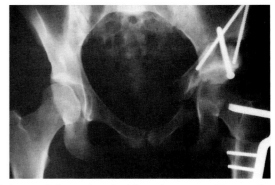

Figure 4. (A) Preoperative radiograph of hip dysplasia involving both the acetabulum and proximal femur in a woman 28 years of age. (B) Anteroposterior postoperative radiograph of same patient after Ganz periacetabular and femoral intertrochanteric osteotomies.

genital hip dysplasia, the acetabulum is hypoplastic, which limits coverage of the femoral head. Surgical correction depends on the age of the patient, degree of deformity, and preservation of articular cartilage. During the last 10 years in the United States, a Ganz or periacetabular osteotomy has gained considerable popularity for adults (Ganz, Klaue, Vinh, & Mast, 1988; Millis, Murphy, & Poss, 1995). Intermediate term success of the procedure has been noted in the European literature, and it has been found that the more severe the arthritis before the osteotomy, the poorer the result (Ganz et al., 1988).

Periacetabular osteotomy can be technically challenging with complications including but not limited to neurovascular injury, intra-articular fracture, under- or overcorrection of the acetabulum position, and nonunion. However, when performed correctly in properly selected patients, the results may last a lifetime and may obviate the need for THA. There are no U.S. statistics on this procedure, which is more popular in Europe. In the United States, the procedure is mainly performed in university medical centers. Large randomized prospective studies will be required before the true effectiveness of this procedure is known.

Postoperative Rehabilitation for Osteotomy

Inpatient therapy in osteotomy progresses quickly because the patients tend to be younger. Length of hospital stay is usually 4 to 5 days. Range of motion (ROM) is limited to either assisted or passive movements. During the procedure, the gluteus medius, gluteus minimus, and the psoas muscles are elevated off the ilium for the posterior bone cuts. The hamstring muscles and reflected head of the rectus muscle are elevated off the ischium for exposure to make the anterior cuts. These muscles are reattached but must be protected for 3 to 6 months. Patients may use a knee sling or a towel to assist supine movement, and they must be taught assisted techniques with the other leg or a strap for transferring from supine to sitting. Sitting is often painful as is knee ROM because of muscular guarding. There may be some positioning and movement restrictions such as no active hip abduction and passive ROM only, and adaptive equipment such as a leg-lifting device may be needed.

Weight-bearing activities begin on postoperative day (POD) 1 or 2. The partial weight-bearing status must continue for 6 or more weeks. A "foot flat" versus "toe touch" gait is recommended. The rationale for this is to protect the osteotomy site by limiting joint forces that are the combined result of muscle contraction and body weight (McLeish & Charnley, 1970). It is estimated that the forces result in a load 1.6 times body weight in the stance phase of slow walking, 2.6 times body weight in single-leg standing, and 3 times body weight in the swing phase of running. Joint forces from muscle contraction alone are quite strong, and it is reported that, during active flexion and extension supine, the forces are greater than during slow walking or with crutch use (Rydell, 1966). Patients are discharged and frequently require home physical therapy or outpatient therapy for ROM. They are not allowed to drive for 12 weeks. Between the 6th and 12th weeks, weight bearing is progressed to full and active motion, and strengthening exercises are progressed through positioning and repetition. Biking and aquatic exercises are undertaken at the discretion of the surgeon. Bony union is usually noted 12 weeks after surgery, at which time the patient is progressed to normal functional activities. Although restrictions may be lifted, patients should be encouraged to continue using a cane until they no longer limp.

Hip Arthroscopy

Indications for hip arthroscopy include labral tears, loose bodies, and infection. Patients with hip dysplasia often have an associated labral tear of the hip (Klaue et al., 1991). In these cases, hip arthroscopy may temporarily alleviate symptoms of the labral tear, such as catching or giving way. However, the long-term solution requires correction of the hip dysplasia through corrective osteotomy. The procedure is technically demanding because of the difficulty of positioning the instruments within the confines of the spherical hip joint. Arthroscopy may be used to treat infection if septicemia is not present. Current usefulness of hip arthroscopy in patients with degenerative hip disease is limited. No good controlled studies exist to support routine arthroscopic debridement of the hip joint as a temporary procedure before joint arthroplasty. However, surgeons who are proficient in hip arthroscopy may consider the procedure for patients who are relatively young with degenerative hip arthritis and loose bodies present on radiographs and a history of mechanical symptoms such as locking or catching in the affected hip. Arthroscopy is a day-surgery procedure for which the patients usually are allowed partial to full weight bearing postoperatively as tolerated. The patient will be encouraged by the physician to begin or resume exercises for motion and strength, and a referral to therapy is indicated if function is limited and pain persists.

Hemiarthroplasty

Use of bipolar and monopolar hemiarthroplasty in hip surgery is usually limited to the treatment of acute femoral neck fractures (Warner et al., 1987). A hemiarthroplasty replaces only one of the two surfaces of the hip joint and usually the femoral side. A hemiarthroplasty is considered a monopolar prosthesis if it articulates directly against the acetabulum. It is bipolar if the femoral prosthetic head moves within another cup that articulates and moves with the acetabulum. Literature indicates that the outcome of bipolar arthroplasty for osteonecrosis of the hip is not as good as for standard THA (Phillips, 1987; Scott, 1984; Scott et al., 1987). In addition, use of a bipolar prosthesis for acetabular reconstruction with morselized grafts (i.e., grafts made from ground bone from the femoral head) has a higher rate of failure, absorption of grafts, and migration of the component compared with fixed acetabular reconstruction (Brien, Warwick, Salvati, Wilson, & Pellicci, 1990; Scott, 1984; Scott et al., 1987; Wilson, Nikpoor, Aliabadi, Poss, & Weissman, 1989). The results of one study recommended the technique only as a salvage procedure in elderly or infirm patients with acetabular deficiency (Brien et al., 1990). In most studies, evaluating the use of bipolar prosthesis for femoral neck fractures, relief of pain, early mobilization, and restoration of function was achieved (Bochner, Pellicci, & Lyden 1988; Warner et al., 1987). Postoperative rehabilitation for this procedure follows the guidelines for THA.

Total Hip Arthroplasty

THA is one of the most common orthopedic procedures in the United States, with more than 200,000 procedures per year at an estimated cost in excess of $2.5 billion per year. Of these, more than two thirds are performed in persons more than 65 years of age. THA offers tremendous benefits, including marked improvement of pain relief, physical function, social interaction, and overall health and sense of well-being (Poss, Brick, Wright, & Sledge, 1988).

Continued controversy regarding the optimal mode of fixation in THA, concerns regarding wear on the polyethylene component that causes particulates to occur in the joint as a cause of osteolysis, and eventual implant failure has had a great effect on choice of implant fixation (Harris, Salzman, Athanasoulis, & Waltman, 1977; Mattingly, Hopson, Kahn, & Giannestras, 1985; Pellicci, Salvati, & Robinson, 1979; Poss, Robertson, & Walker, 1988; Poss, Brick, et al., 1988; Rimac, Wright, & McGill, 1986). More recent use of robotics and computer-assisted designed implants for improved fit and fill of the femoral canal will require longer-term clinical follow-up before advantages are realized. The widespread use of these technological advances may be impeded by cost-containment measures in health care.

Current and future success of THA will be determined objectively on a physician-derived evaluation of prosthetic function (e.g., ROM, function, radiographs) and subjectively by patient-derived evaluation and satisfaction with the outcome. An international clinical evaluation system to determine the success of THA is being developed so that information between institutions and countries can be critically examined and compared (Mueller, Sledge, & Poss, 1990).

Cemented THA

Sir John Charnley introduced low-friction hip arthroplasty in 1962. Since then, many of his original concepts and techniques serve as the basis for THA, including the use of cement for component fixation (Figure 5; Charnley, 1972). However, many of the same problems with cement fixation persist, and the most common complication of cemented THA remains aseptic loosening. Earlier reports on 10-year follow-up of implants that used early cement techniques revealed higher femoral than acetabular loosening occurring radiographically in one third of patients. Longer-term studies (more than 20 years) documented the over-

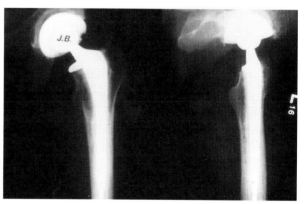

Figure 5. Anteroposterior (left) and lateral radiograph (right) of hybrid THA with cemented femoral stem and uncemented acetabular cup.

all durability of the Charnley implant with cement fixation, especially in older patients. Failure of femoral stems tends to be linear and averages around 1% per year during the first two decades. Acetabular cement fixation is less durable with higher cup revision rates during the same period (7–16% revision rate) (Charnley, 1972; Harris & McGann, 1986; Pellicci et al., 1979; Poss, Robertson, et al., 1988.

Newer cementing techniques (including the use of a femoral plug, retrograde filling of the femur with a cement gun, pulsatile lavage of the bone interstices, vacuum mixing of the cement to reduce porosity, and pressurization of the cement) are expected to improve results of cemented prostheses (Burke, Gates, & Harris, 1984; Rimac et al., 1986). Proponents of cemented femoral stems point out the excellent results with a cemented Charnley stem even with early cement techniques, including finger packing of the cement. Using newer techniques has led to reports of vastly superior performance of the femoral component. However, longer-term data will be required to substantiate these results (Harris et al., 1977; Roberts, Poss, & Kelley, 1986; Russotti, Coventry, & Stauffer, 1988).

Cement is believed to form an excellent proximal barrier to polyethylene debris, which has the potential to cause diffuse osteolysis around the femoral implant. In addition, immediate unprotected weight bearing can be allowed with a lower incidence of thigh pain compared with uncemented stems. Newer techniques of prosthetic fixation should be compared with results obtained with modern cement techniques. A drawback to cement fixation is the difficulty in removing the prothesis if a revision is necessary.

Uncemented THA

Clinical failures of cemented THA stimulated investigations into alternative fixation methods. The technique of uncemented THA involves surgically implanting femoral or acetabular prostheses into bone and relies on osseous integration (bone growing into the femoral stem) to obtain a mechanical interlock between the prosthesis and bone (Figure 6). Tissue ingrowth occurs between 3 and 6 months, with bone remodeling continuing after that time.

There are two methods to achieve osseous integration. Advocates of the press-fit technique believe there is more uniform transfer of stresses to proximal bone than with porous coating. Those favoring porous coating question the long-term durability and stability of press-fit fixation (Poss, Brick, et al., 1988; Poss, Robertson, et al., 1988. More recently, ceramics (most notably hydroxyapatite) have been applied to some porous-coated stems to enhance the potential of bony ingrowth. Early clinical follow-up appears promising; however, further clinical and biomechanical research will be required to determine the effectiveness of this treatment.

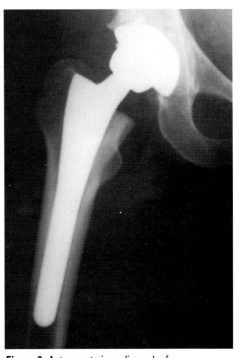

Figure 6. Anteroposterior radiograph of uncemented THA.

Complications of THA

Infection is one of the most serious complications of THA. The incidence of sepsis is approximately 1% during the lifetime of the prosthesis, with approximately half of the infections believed to begin at the time of operation (Fitzgerald, Nolan, & Ilstrup, 1977; Maderazo, Judson, & Pasternak, 1988). Preoperative antibiotics have been found to be the most important element of reducing acute total joint sepsis. However, a large prospective double-blind study found no difference in the infection rate when using antibiotics for 1 day (cefuroxime) versus 3 days (cefazolin) postoperatively. In addition, a major decrease in infection rate has been noted with the use of ultra-clean air, body exhaust suites, and ultraviolet (UV) light. A recent comparison of UV light to ultra-clean air enclosure revealed the UV light to be 34 times less expensive and just as effective in preventing infection in THA (Berg, Bergman, & Hoborn, 1991; Berg-Perier, Cederblad, & Persson, 1992). Critics of UV light point out the need for protective clothing and the risk of exposure for staff members and the patient. There are no international guidelines for occupational exposure to UV radiation (National Institute for Occupational Safety and Health, 1972).

Surgical management of a deep prosthetic infection may involve removal of the components with debridement. Debridement may be a one-stage revision involving removal of old components and reimplantation of new components with administration of systemic antibiotics or a two-stage reimplantation with removal of components followed by 6 weeks of antibiotics and reimplantation at a later date. A resection of the femoral head or removal of the femoral prothesis without reimplantation is called a *girdlestone procedure* or a *resection arthroplasty*. Management decisions are determined by the age and overall health of the patient, the type and sensitivity of the organism, and whether the infection is acute or chronic. The use of antibiotic-impregnated cement in both one- and two-stage procedures can improve the salvage rate in both procedures.

Dislocation rates after THA vary from 1% to 10% (Poss, Brick, et al., 1988). Usually instability after THA is related to malpositioning of the cup or stem. However, other associated factors include previous surgery, weak abductor, impingement, and surgical approach. Most hip dislocations occur within the first month of surgery. The incidence of recurrent dislocation is less in those who dislocate within 1 month of surgery than in those who dislocate within 3 months of surgery. Revision surgery for recurrent hip instability includes revising one or both components, increasing leg length and offset, using an elevated liner, and trochanteric advancement. When the cause of instability is clearly identifiable and corrected, the success rate is about 70% and drops to less than 50% if no identifiable cause can be determined.

Soft-tissue repair during THA includes anatomical reapproximation of tissue planes with suture. In addition, we reattach the short external rotators—the piriformis and conjoined tendon and posterior capsule—to the greater trochanter through drill holes with strong nonabsorbable sutures. Most researchers believe the technique may provide for greater hip stability postoperatively. In addition, the technique may prevent formation of excess scar tissue around the hip joint as is sometimes noted when complete capsulectomy is performed. Since using this technique, we have observed a decrease in hip dislocation rate. Hip dislocation precautions are continued for 12 weeks postoperatively.

Other complications of THA include deep vein thrombosis (DVT), pulmonary embolus, periprosthetic fracture, loosening of the components, and formation of heterotopic bone. DVT is the most frequent complication after THA in patients 39 years of age or older (Paiement, Schutzer, Wessinger, & Harris, 1992). When prophylaxis is not used, 40% to 70% of patients develop DVT (Beisaw, Comerota, & Groth, 1988; Evarts & Feil, 1971; Harris & McGann, 1986; Johnson, Carmichael, Almond, & Loynes, 1978; Rogers, Walsh, & Marden, 1978). One of the greatest fears of DVT is that it may lead to pulmonary embolus, which is one of the most serious complications of THA. The risk of clinically significant pulmonary embolus is higher with proximal vein thrombosis. In patients undergoing THA without prophylaxis, the rate of nonfatal pulmonary embolus ranges from 3.2% to 16.9% and the rate of fatal pulmonary embolus from 0% to 6.7% (Berquist,

Efsing, Hallbook, & Hedlund, 1979; Charnley, 1972; Rothermal, Weissinger, & Stinchfield, 1973; Schondorf & Hey, 1976; Wolf, Hozack, Balderston, Booth, & Rothman, 1992).

Heterotopic ossification (HO) occurs from noncirculating connective tissue cells that have the potential to differentiate and form bone. The radiographic rate of HO after hip surgery is between 8% and 90% (Ayers, Evarts, & Parkinson, 1986). A higher incidence is noted for patients who are men (approximately twice the incidence than for women), have had bilateral procedures, have a previous history of HO, have had revision hip surgery, and are more than 60 years of age. The incidence of symptomatic HO after THA ranges from 1% to 33%. Prophylactic treatment includes nonsteroidal anti-inflammatory medication or radiation therapy. Radiation treatment should be given within 3 days of surgery with shielding of uncemented implants and trochanteric osteotomies. Recent protocols with single-fraction 700-cGy radiation therapy has been shown to be effective in lowering the incidence of HO (Ayers et al., 1986). There may be local pain during the formation and maturation process of HO, which may take up to 18 months. After this time, the motion will be limited but painless. The HO can be surgically excised if there is a major loss of motion.

Postoperative Rehabilitation for THA

Pain relief and improvement in function are the goals of the surgeon, the patient, and the rehabilitation team.

Preoperative Care

Because many THA surgeries are elective, the health care team may have the opportunity to examine the patient preoperatively and if so should begin the evaluation, education, and discharge plans (Ganz & Viellion, 1996). (See chapter 1 for a discussion on preoperative education.) Table 2 lists suggested topics for group patient education programs.

Preoperative physical therapy and occupational therapy evaluations are often a luxury unless they are included in a preoperative education program. During a preoperative visit, self-reported health status indices and functional evaluations may be obtained. These forms are extremely useful outcome measures, and the data should be collected preoperatively and at designated postoperative intervals.

Table 2. Topics for a Preoperative Education for Patients Planning a THA

Anatomy of normal and diseased joint (skeletal models and illustrations)
Disease process
Surgical procedure in nonmusical terms
Prosthetic designs
Precautions and the rationales
Postoperative positioning and equipment (intravenous line, catheter, suspension)
Pain management
Postoperative exercise program and rationale
Gait training with the ambulatory device and explanation of weight-bearing status
Considerations for discharge
Questions and answers
Reassurance

Many orthopedic departments have computerized outcome data registries and use instruments that have been agreed to by a broad consensus of surgeons. The Medical Outcomes Study Short Form (SF-36) is a general health status index (Ware & Sherbourne, 1992); see the Appendix at the end of the book), and the Western Ontario MacMaster Universities Osteoarthritis Index (WOMAC) is a specific hip and knee questionnaire that evaluates degree of difficulty, pain, and stiffness (Bellamy, Buchanan, Goldsmith, Campbell, & Still, 1988; see Appendix 2 in chapter 6 of this book).

The trend in health care is reengineering and work redesign with the emphasis on outcomes, not tasks (Hammer & Campy, 1993). As with other medical and surgical hospital admissions, the reengineering trend is toward a uniform interdisciplinary evaluation without duplication of process. Each professional will ask questions in his or her domain and complete relevant sections of the evaluation, which decreases repeated questioning of the patient and streamlines the process. A patient only needs to be asked once if there are stairs in the house and what are the current medications. Table 3 lists subjective and objective components for a preoperative evaluation.

Although the physical and emotional benefits of THA are well documented (Erickson & Perkins, 1994; Quinet & Winter, 1992), rehabilitation parameters, programming, and outcomes are not consistent or standardized (Enlow, Shields, Smith, Leo, & Miller, 1996; Platt, Hahn, Kessler, & McCarthy, 1986; Zuckerman, Kummer, & Frankel, 1994). Earlier discharge from the acute care facility has required practitioners to shift their emphasis to earlier initiation of treatment focusing on achievement of functional goals with discharge to home as independently as possible, where therapy can be continued or progressed on an outpatient or home health care basis. Discharge planning optimally should begin before surgery. Important factors to consider that influence discharge to home include, but are not limited to, level of in-home assistance, functional ADL status, and cognitive abilities.

Intraoperative care. Patients who receive oral steroids routinely will be given intravenous steroids during surgery to prevent the possibility of an adrenal crisis. Oral steroids will again be given when the patient can tolerate an oral diet. These patients tend to have little subcutaneous tissue, which makes their skin vulnerable to injury. It is wise to use extra padding on the operating table to prevent potential skin problems. A pneumatic boot should be placed on the down-positioned leg. Laminar air flow is used in most operating rooms to prevent or lessen infections. Prophylactic intravenous antibiotics are given before the start of surgery and are continued for 24 to 48 hr.

Postoperative care pathways. Care pathways that have been developed for routine THA patients describe medical, surgical, and rehabilitative interventions from the date of surgery to discharge. The length of stay ranges from 4 to 7 days for an uncomplicated single-joint arthroplasty. Appendix 1 is a sample care pathway for patients and family members from Brigham and Women's Hospital (Boston, MA). See Appendix 2, the Multidisciplinary Documentation Total Hip DRG 209 form from the University of Pittsburgh Medical Center, St. Margaret Hospital (Pittsburgh, PA).

Positioning and Skin Care

Postoperative positioning is decided on the basis of the surgeon's philosophy and the hospital's preference. The most common variations are sling-pillow suspension with or without Buck's traction, an abductor pillow, or conventional pillows (Figure 7). Antiembolic stockings and external sequential pneumatic leg-compression devices may likewise be used (Kaempffe, Lifeso, & Meinking, 1991).

Another consideration for the patient with multiple joint involvement is positioning for rest after surgery, as well as for rehabilitation. Many patients are not able to lie flat because of spinal involvement such as in spinal stenosis, ankylosing spondylitis, longstanding postural limitations, or hip and knee flexion contractures. The goal of positioning is comfort while maintaining as anatomically correct a position as possible. Depending on the surgical approach and protocol, the patient may

Table 3. Rehabilitation Evaluation

Subjective pain
- Type, location, onset, duration, intensity
- Pattern (evening or day, before or after activity, sleep or at rest, weight bearing ornon-weight bearing)
- How does pain limit function?

History of previous injury
History of arthritis
- Which joints are involved?
- Previous interventions and surgeries
- Upper-extremity involvement that would limit use of ambulatory devices

ROM and strength

Medications

Radiographic and laboratory results

Pertinent medical history including comorbid conditions that may affect recovery (e.g., COPD, CAD, fibromyalgia, diabetes, and sensory deficits such as paraesthesias, loss of proprioception, visual or auditory loss)

Environmental and social situation
- Is the plan to return home or to another location after surgery?
- Barriers at home (e.g., location of bathroom, bedroom, and kitchen)
- Stairs with or without rails
- Assistance at home (e.g., cooking, cleaning, shopping)
- Work situation and job physical demands
- Leisure activities

Functional evaluation
- Ability to perform lower-body self-care
- Ability to perform transfers
- Are assistive and or ambulatory devices already being used?
- Are joint protection principles being used?

Cognitive evaluation
- Identification of issues that may impair learning and full participation in the postoperative program (e.g., memory, disorientation, judgment of safety)
- Education—What has been retained from previous interventions?
- Patient goals and expectations

Physical evaluation
- Posture and how it will affect postoperative program
- Skin (nodules, fragility)
- Discrepancy in leg length
- Gait
- ROM (active and passive)
- Flexion, extension (Thomas Test position), abduction, adduction, internal rotation, external rotation in flexion and or extension
- Strength: isometric resistance to determine integrity of muscles (a lower quadrant screen to identify deficits that would compromise rehabilitation—strength is often limited by pain, not specific muscle weakness)
- Neurological screening of the lower extremity

Function
- Transfer
  —Supine to sit to supine, and sit to stand and sit
  —How well are hands used?
- Ambulation
  —Usual and maximum distance or time
  —Devices used? Gait pattern?
  —Stairs (how many? is a rail present?)

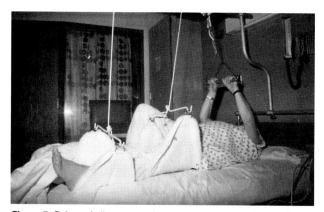

Figure 7. Balanced sling suspension and trapeze set up for a patient after THA.

be allowed to lie on his or her side to rest. Lying on the operative side is preferable because it lessens the chance of dislocation because the hip is in a neutral position. The patient, however, usually cannot tolerate this in the early postoperative period, so lying on the unoperative side may be allowed as long as the top leg remains in neutral alignment. This usually requires a few firm pillows or an abductor pillow. Patients with severe contractures generally report greater comfort when in sling-pillow suspension because the strain is lessened on the tight structures. It is important to prevent further deformity. Gentle stretching of tight tissues such as the hip adductors and the hip flexors can be initiated and must be continued and intensified after discharge.

The patient who cannot lie flat may need to be positioned with pillows. Towel rolls can be used under the neck or low back, and consideration should be given to areas that may develop pressure sores from the supine position. Heels need particular attention in patients who have knee contractures. The patient should be allowed to bring his or her pillow to the hospital if it will facilitate position and comfort.

The patient is usually catheterized for the first 1 to 2 days. An intravenous catheter will be in place until it is no longer needed for intravenous antibiotics or patient-controlled anesthesia. Postoperative pain is initially managed by either an epidural block, a patient-controlled analgesia pump, or intramuscular injection. On the first or second day, the patient may be transferred to oral analgesics as needed. Because the potential for thrombosis exists, the patient will usually receive some form of anticoagulant therapy—warfarin, aspirin, or enoxaparin.

A surgical drain, if used, will be in place for 1 to 2 days postoperatively. About 200 to 500 ml of drainage is expected during the first 24 hr. Meticulous attention is given to skin care, particularly in this population, which tends to be older and has other chronic disease or musculoskeletal problems.

A nonhealing wound may be indicative of an infection or of the patient's poor preoperative nutritional and immunological status. According to Hanssen, Osmon, and Nelson (1996), a total lymphocyte count of less than $1500/mm^3$ and an albumin level of less than 35 g/L are indicative of a greater potential for a nonhealing wound. Ideally, if these problems are discovered preoperatively, nutritional supplements can be prescribed and surgery delayed until these indicators are in a more desirable range for good wound healing.

Maintaining hip precautions is not only the responsibility of the patient but also for nursing and therapy staff members. Not seeking assistance when transferring a patient, trying to transfer too quickly without the patient's cooperation, or not having the immediate bedside environment set up properly are potential sources of movements that can cause dislocation. The telephone, call bell, tray table, and so forth should be on the side of the arthroplasty to minimize the chance of dislocation from combinations of adduction and internal rotation and from twisting.

Dislocation Precautions

The surgical approach and the patient's mental status are two variables influencing the precautions. These precautions must be adhered to for at least 6 to 8 weeks for soft-tissue healing. At 3 months, most patients have developed sufficient muscle control to dispense with the precautions, but the surgeon should give final clearance. The patient should ask about the precautions if he or she is not told specifically. The following patient guidelines are influenced by institutional and regional philosophy. There are no universal dislocation precautions, but it is generally agreed that a combination of motions is more likely to cause a dislocation rather than just a single motion (i.e., 90° of flexion). See Table 4 for a list of patient instructions. When the procedure is a revision arthroplasty, the precautions may be different and more extensive and should be documented by the surgeon. Often, in revision surgery, the greater trochanter is osteotomized to aid in the removal of the prosthesis. Its reattachment must be protected, so weight bearing and activities of the gluteus medius are often limited.

Bed Activities

When the patient is turned in bed, the operative leg should always remain in neutral or abduction, and the entire length of the leg should be supported when turning toward the unoperative side. A fracture bed pan is preferred versus the standard-size bed pan because it is smaller and requires less movement and effort from the patient. If possible, the patient flexes the nonoperative hip and knee and attempts "to bridge" while using the trapeze to lift the pelvis safely on and off the bed pan. If the patient's upper extremities do not allow for the use of the trapeze, then the patient partially rolls toward the operative side, and the bed pan is placed in from the side.

Table 4. Patient Instructions

Anterior surgical approach (patient instructions)
- Do not cross legs.
- Do not lie on your stomach.
- Do not extend your leg behind you.
- Do not twist on the leg when you are standing on it.
- When side-lying, use two to three pillows between your legs.
- When lying on your back, separate your legs with pillows.
- Avoid combination motions of flexion, abduction, external rotation.

Posterior–posterolateral approach (patient instructions)
- Do not cross legs.
- Do not bend hip greater than 90°.
- Do not reach for low objects.
- When side-lying, use two to three pillows between your legs.
- When lying on your back, separate your legs with pillows.
- Avoid combination motion of abduction, flexion, and external rotation.

Physical Therapy Transfers: Gait Training

In the early postoperative stages, it is best for the patient to transfer in and out of bed on the side of the surgery. If bilateral procedures are performed, then transfers should be to the side in which the patient can perform them more safely. Again, after bilateral procedures, the patient should use additional caution.

A ladder attached to a bar at the end of the bed may be needed during the first few transfers as an assist to long sitting and mobility to the edge of the bed. This ladder will aid bathing and linen changing. Patients should progress from the ladder as soon as possible, or they will become dependent on it. On elbows or hands is the next step to independent bed mobility. These positions offer better control to the leg than moving from a supine position.

If the patient's feet do not touch the floor, then a foot stool should be used to maintain the hip in proper alignment. An unsupported hip usually will fall into adduction and internal rotation because of weakness. If a foot stool is used, then the entire bed must be elevated for comfort and to avoid excessive flexion.

The epidural catheter must be removed before transferring. A low hematocrit is not an automatic contraindication to the mobilization of the patient. Hematocrit levels frequently will drift down 3 to 4 points for 2 to 3 days and should be monitored by the medical staff members. Most patients will have orthostatic hypotension the first few times out of bed, so they should sit for a few minutes before transferring. In some hospitals, the nursing staff members will have the responsibility for getting the patient up the first time.

Most patients will sit on the side of the bed on POD 1. Some may transfer out of bed. Sitting for longer than 30 min should be discouraged no matter what the patient requests. It is always more difficult to transfer back into bed because the hip may be painful and the patient tired.

It may be necessary to provide extra cushions in chairs and wheelchairs for added seat height and to elevate the bed and mat to make standing up easier. The cushions and increased height will lessen the degree of flexion when sitting. Whether elevated chairs and toilet seats are needed, it is important to stress adherence to the precautions during all transfers. Rocking movements or momentum should be avoided because they can lead to unpredictable motions at the hip that may cause dislocation. There are numerous adaptations for elevating chairs, and there are higher designed chairs with or without built-in footrests, but the latter can be quite costly and should be considered only if the problem will not resolve with rehabilitation.

Most patients receive therapy in their rooms and in the corridors. Some facilities that have transport services provide therapy in the rehabilitation department if the patient can tolerate sitting in a wheelchair. Transportation aides must be trained in safe transfer techniques and should ask for assistance from the nursing staff members. Ambulation is begun either with a walker or with the parallel bars.

Patients who have joint involvement of the shoulders, elbows, hands, and wrists are often unable to tolerate the stress of using an ambulatory device. Standard crutches, canes, and walkers not only require upper-extremity strength but also sufficient wrist and elbow extension to allow weight bearing. When there is insufficient motion or polyarticular or upper-extremity arthritis, platform crutches are recommended. These have rigid or movable hand pieces with forearm troughs for the weight-bearing surface. A teaching session is usually required to learn how to maneuver them, and most patients have difficulty with balance and with advancing each crutch. Patients are taught to advance the crutch with the strap and to only direct the placement of it with the hand piece. The patient should not pick up the crutch with the hand piece.

A platform attachment can be added to axillary crutches, and, if attachments are not readily available or are uncomfortable, they can be fabricated out of wood or Orthoplast™ (Johnson & Johnson Professional, Inc., Raynham, MA). When platform attachments are added to a walker, the walker can become quite heavy. It may be necessary to add wheels to the front end, which enables the patient to push rather than lift the device (Figure 8). Occasionally, a custom-style crutch attachment may be needed for the patient with severe contractures (elbow contracture greater than 90°) or for the young person with juvenile rheumatoid arthritis who is concerned about the restrictive and cosmetic limitations of a walker.

Hand grips and weight-bearing surfaces of the ambulatory device must be considered. A wider, flat surface allows weight bearing on the palm as opposed to the metacarpophalangeal joints (Figure 8). Grips that can be rotated to accommodate limitations in supination are more comfortable. Padding can be added to provide an increase in diameter for easier grasping, cushioning to bony prominences, and increased shock absorption. Sometimes hand splints are needed to promote adequate joint protection for the hands during ambulation. For patients with thumb adduction contractures, it may be necessary to make the grip narrower by removing the plastic grip and covering the post with thin foam or moleskin.

After providing the patient with a device modified to his or her particular situation, it is important to continue to monitor the patient closely because stress may shift from one joint to another joint, or pain may occur in the postoperative joint because the patient is unable to bear sufficient weight on the upper extremities to protect that joint. Walking may have to be limited until the patient is better able to tolerate upper-extremity weight bearing or until the restrictions are lifted.

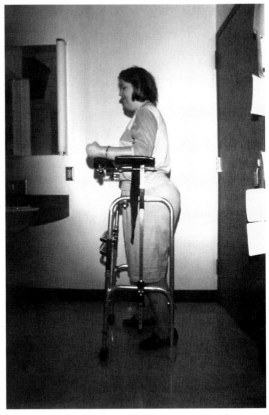

Figure 8. Platform walking aids are recommended for patients with RA and hand impairment. A platform walker is often used during the first postoperative days. Most patients are progressed to crutches before discharge.

Simultaneous arthroplasties (performed under the same anesthesia) are being performed more frequently than in the past when they were staged 5 to 14 days apart. There are no statistically significant differences in outcome regarding staging of procedures. Ankylosing spondylitis is one disease for which simultaneous procedures are performed. It is difficult to intubate these patients or to place a spinal catheter because of the ossification of the ligaments, so, from a medical point of view, one anesthesia is preferred. From a nursing and rehabilitation perspective, the first few days are labor intensive, but it is easier for the patient to progress because both hips have increased movement.

In ankylosing spondylitis patients, the rehabilitation staff members must remember that just because the joints have potential for greater motion, the ability to move in bed, transfer, and stand up straighter may not change greatly because of a kyphotic posture or rigidity of the spine. Balance should always be considered. Encourage the patient to stand tall, but do not force a posture that may be impossible to safely achieve and maintain.

Weight-bearing status varies with the surgeon's protocol, prosthetic type and fixation, bony integrity, whether the procedure is a primary arthroplasty or a revision, and complications such as intraoperative fractures.

A general rule has been that patients with cemented prostheses usually can bear weight (with a device) as tolerated. Weight-bearing guidelines, therefore, are necessary to protect the soft tissues and minimize pain. Patients with press-fit, uncemented components must remain touch-down to partial weight bearing for at least 6 weeks to protect and allow for tissue ingrowth into the prosthesis. Touch-down is calculated at 0 to 30% of body weight and partial weight bearing up to 50%. A bathroom scale is the least expensive method to instruct the patient in weight-bearing restrictions. Pressure screening devices and boots are available.

Exercise Planning

Exercise programs for patients after THA are not clearly defined or proven effective (Givens-Heiss et al., 1992; Krebs, Elbaum, Riley, Hodge, & Mann, 1991; Mattson, Bronstrom, & Linnarsson, 1990; Shih, Du, Lin, & Wu, 1994; Strickland et al., 1992). Often the approach taken to exercise prescription has been decided on the basis of tradition, practitioner and surgeon preference, and patient level of pain and functioning. In developing an exercise prescription, the patient's needs must be considered and how he or she may differ from the norm must be established in the critical pathway. Consider the following:

- Will the patient be able to protect weight bearing?
- Will the patient be able to use an ambulatory device?
- Are the upper extremities and uninvolved lower extremity strong enough?
- What effects will the patient's deformities have on rehabilitation?
- Are there any other comorbidities that will affect activity?
- Are the patient's bones osteoporotic?
- Were there any operative complications (e.g., femur fracture, nerve injury)?

- Was the trochanter osteotomized?
- What was the surgical approach, and what are the precautions due to the prosthesis and fixation?

Exercise prescription commonly consists of an exercise type, number of repetitions, times per day, and instructions about position and technique. Most important is education about why the exercises are to be performed and how they will benefit the patient in the long term. A patient who understands the benefits is more likely to comply with the program. Table 5 lists exercise by purpose and position.

On POD 1, quadriceps and gluteal isometrics, active assisted hip ROM, and exercises for the other joints are begun. The exercises progress until discharge, at which time the patient can do sitting and standing active exercises. Progression beyond that point is done in the home or at a rehabilitation or outpatient facility. Prone lying may begin during hospitalization, but the focus is on transfers, ambulation, and function. Biking, which at one time was routine treatment in THA, is seldom done for motion, and, if allowed, begins during the strengthening phases of rehabilitation, 6 to 8 weeks postoperatively.

Exercise philosophy and controversies. Participating in exercise for both motion and strength used to be considered a prerequisite for ambulation. The patient would do bed exercises for a few days before ambulation began. This has changed with the advancement in protocols, and now old and new research is used in rehabilitation planning. As previously mentioned, there are more forces on the hip joint during supine exercises than in ambulation (Rydell, 1966). More recent research in joint compression forces during maximal voluntary isometrics, although still preliminary and not yet generalized to a broad population, suggested that this type of exercise places a greater force across the hip joint with an endoprosthesis than in full weight bearing (Krebs et al., 1991). There is ongoing research on acetabular pressures (i.e., the measurement of stress in a newly replaced hip joint).

Table 5. Postoperative Exercise Prescription for THA

Purpose	Exercise	Position
Prevent respiratory problems	Deep breathing, coughing	Supine, sitting
Prevent blood clots	Ankle pumps, ROM other joints	Supine, sitting
Increase ROM	Active assisted ROM, with a sling, human assistance, positioning	Supine, prone
Increase strength	Active ROM	Supine, sitting, standing
	Isometric exercise	Supine, sitting, standing, sidelying
	Open-chain exercise: sitting and total knee extension	Standing, sitting
	(Progress with increased repetitions or use of light weights or Thera-band™)	
	Closed-chain exercise: wall slides, biking, gym equipment	

The concept of peak acetabular pressure has yet to be fully understood, and data from these studies will help determine the effectiveness and appropriateness of specific exercise programs (Krebs et al., 1991). These same studies suggest that, during exercise, the patient may have some control of force across the hip joint by the amount of effort exerted during the exercise.

Protocols vary widely in terms of straight leg raising (SLR). Studies suggest that SLR may be too stressful because of the long lever arm length of the leg that results in greater torque about the hip joint, and others suggest that SLR is actually less stressful than isometric abduction (Givens-Heiss et al., 1992; Krebs et al., 1991; Mattson et al., 1990; Shih, Du, Lin, & Wu, 1994; Strickland et al., 1992).

There is no consensus on the use of resistance for strengthening other than it should not be done until the soft tissue is adequately healed, which is at approximately 6 to 8 weeks. Some surgeons believe that functional activities are sufficient for strengthening, and others encourage the use of light free weights, Theraband™ (Hygenic Corp., Akron, OH), and exercise equipment. The decision is made on the basis of the surgical procedure and the activity demands to which the patient will return.

It is now documented that weakness after THA may continue for up to 2 years, even when the patient exhibits a normal gait (National Institutes of Health, 1994). It has been further shown that lower-extremity weakness is a major risk factor for falls in elderly persons (Brander, Stulber, & Chang, 1993). Weakness in the hip abductors especially can change joint forces and lead to an unstable hip joint (Shih, Du, Lin, & Wu, 1994). Neumann (1996) studied hip abductor muscle forces in persons with hip prostheses as they carry varying loads, and he concurred. The larger the load on the contralateral side, the greater the demand on the prothesis joint, possibly increasing the chances of loosening. Neumann (1996) recommended caution in the early stages of rehabilitation, particularly with cementless hips, and recommended providing instructions and alternative strategies for carrying heavy items after ambulation aids are dispensed with.

A patient with weak hip abductors can either have a Trendelenburg gait, whereby the pelvis on the contralateral side drops with weight bearing on the weak hip, or a compensated pattern in which the torso is shifted over the weak hip during stance. Both gait patterns can be fatiguing and place greater stress on the joint and musculature. Therefore, it is imperative that the patient be instructed on a progressive gluteus medius strengthening program. When the patient is able to exercise in the standing position, proprioception and balance can be incorporated into the program.

Occupational Therapy

Occupational therapy will likely begin on POD 1, especially if preoperative evaluation and training did not occur. Depending on tolerance, the first visit may include bed or chair transfer and, if able, review of the use of lower-extremity assistive devices. From POD 2 until discharge, occupational therapy will provide retraining in ADL that emphasizes the integration of hip precautions in the following areas:

- bed and chair transfers
- toilet transfers
- bathtub and shower transfers
- lower-body bathing

- lower-body dressing
- car transfers (review procedure)

Family members and caregivers should be instructed in these techniques. See the list of resources at the end of the chapter for a list of catalogs of assistive devices and alternative techniques that may be needed. The Abledata database on the Internet is an excellent resource for equipment that may not be available in regular catalogs (www.abledata.com).

In addition, other areas of ADL are addressed if they are problematic. For instance, home management tasks and appropriate alternative techniques should be addressed if the patient will be responsible for those activities after discharge. Likewise, the occupational therapy practitioner may need to address sexual positioning, work activities, and leisure activities and make appropriate recommendations for modifications to allow the patient to do these activities safely (Melvin, 1989).

Sports and exercises that are gliding in nature such as biking are safer than impact sports. Leisure activities that should be avoided include running, football, soccer, singles racquet sports, basketball, volleyball, and hockey. Recommended sports are swimming, walking, golfing, sailing, and occasionally doubles racquet sports. Skiing and horseback riding are usually discouraged because of the injuries that can occur from a fall (McGory, Stuart, & Sim, 1995).

Home Recommendations

Bed positioning and transfer

- Generally, keep a pillow between the thighs as a reminder to maintain an abducted position. Do not be fooled—a pillow will not prevent unwanted motion. If precautions are strict because of an unstable hip or an agitated patient, then a firm abducted pillow should be strapped between the legs.
- After achieving a seated or semiseated position, move the leg closest to the edge of the bed over the side. Maintain it in a neutral rotation. Turn the entire body as the remaining leg is adducted to neutral and moved over the edge.
- Raise the bed on blocks if it is too low to stand up from or when the hips would be in greater than 90° of flexion while sitting.
- When returning to bed, sit on the edge one third to one half the way down from the head.
- Nightstand, telephone, and so forth should be on the operated side.

Sitting

- When sitting, the knees should be at the same level or slightly lower than the hips.
- Sit in firm seats with arm supports; avoid low soft chairs, sofas, and recliners.
- An elevated seat may temporarily be needed as well as a raised toilet seat to prevent hip flexion greater than 90° and to increase the ease of standing up.
- Avoid crossing the legs or sitting with the legs internally rotated.

Bathing

- Do not try to sit on the bottom of the bathtub. Use a commercially available transfer shower stool with a hand-held shower or long-handled sponge to reach the lower extremities.

Walk-in showers make entering and exiting easier, but, whatever the setting, adequate grab bars for support are needed.

Dressing

- Get dressed from a firmly seated position.
- Dress the operated leg first, and reverse the procedure for undressing.
- Use a dressing stick to start the slacks and underwear over the operated leg first. Then, put in the unoperated leg and use the stick to pull the clothing up to the knees. Stand with the ambulatory device, and pull the clothes up to the waist.
- Use a sock or stocking aid for putting socks or stockings on and the dressing stick to assist with getting them off below the knee level.
- Wear supportive slip-on shoes or insert elastic laces into tie shoes. A long shoe horn is important for avoiding excessive bending.

Car transfer

- To get into a car, back up to the seat. Slowly sit down on the seat with the operated leg extended. Move the buttocks further into the seat and slowly turn the whole body into the car, carefully avoiding excessive hip flexion and adduction. If it is difficult to move the buttocks on the seat, place a plastic bag on the seat, which will aid in sliding.
- Enter the car standing on ground level; standing on a curb makes the car seat even lower to the ground.

Home management

- Store frequently used items within reach that does not require bending, and use long-handled reachers to retrieve objects from the floor or from low shelves.
- If ambulating with a walker, attach a multipocketed walker bag or use a waist pack to carry small items.
- Use long-handled sponges, mops, and dusters to prevent excessive flexion.

Patient and Family Education for Discharge

The rapid changes in health care reimbursement have encouraged earlier hospital discharges either to the patient's home or to a subacute facility. This decreased length of stay has necessitated patient education to emphasize "survival skills" at home to be followed by further teaching either in home health care or at follow-up visits to the surgeon. The survival skills include how to do self-care with the appropriate hip precautions, home exercise programs, signs and symptoms of infection and hip dislocation, and knowledge of medications, especially if the patient is being discharged while taking an anticoagulant. In some institutions, it is the case manager's responsibility to make follow-up calls after discharge. In other facilities, early telephone follow-up is coordinated through the surgeon's office or the primary nurse.

One area of patient education often neglected is sexual activity. The patient is instructed that he or she should take a dependent position for 3 to 6 months postoperatively (Smeltzer & Bare, 1992). Patients must think through their positioning during sexual intercourse and make sure that they are maintaining their hip precautions at all times.

Discharge Instructions

A written exercise sheet with the precautions described in simple terms should be provided along with guidelines for wound care and pain medication use. Written guidelines for the prophylactic use of antibiotics before procedures such as tooth extraction or colonoscopy should likewise be provided (Hanssen et al., 1996; Smeltzer & Bare, 1992).

Arthrodesis

Hip arthrodesis has fallen out of favor with patients since the advent of THA, and the authors cannot recall the last time they performed or treated a hip fusion. The advantages of THA include the ability to maintain a normal gait, ROM, and a modified but active lifestyle. However, these advantages must be balanced against poorer clinical results long term and the probable need for multiple revisions during the lifetime of a younger patient.

Fusion of the hip is usually reserved for the younger patient (less than 40 years of age). To be a candidate for a fusion, the patient must have a normal lumbosacral spine, ipsilateral knee, and contralateral hip. Indications include unilateral posttraumatic or septic arthritis in an otherwise young healthy patient who wants to remain unrestricted in activities. In addition, younger patients with severe developmental arthropathy or arthritis secondary to avascular necrosis of the femoral head should be considered for hip arthrodesis (Figure 9).

A successful hip fusion will allow the patient to return to full activities, including heavy labor. The ideal position for fusion is 20° to 25° of hip flexion, neutral adduction, and neutral rotation. On gait analysis, the average walking speed with a hip arthrodesis is 84% of normal, and the mean oxygen consumption is approximately 32% greater than normal and represents a gait efficiency of 53%. Several studies reporting the long-term results of hip arthrodesis have documented a high patient satisfaction with good pain relief, acceptable function, and ability to return to work (Sponseller, McBeath, & Perpich, 1984).

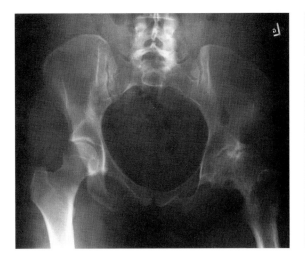 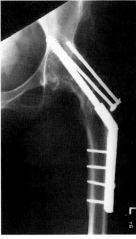

Figure 9. (A) Preoperative anteroposterior radiograph of pelvis demonstrating severe developmental OA in a woman 33 years of age with a previous history of slipped capital femoral epiphysis. (B) Postoperative anteroposterior radiograph of same patient treated with hip arthrodesis.

Patients are in a hip spica cast for 10 to 12 weeks, and weight bearing is 50%. During hospitalization, a fracture pan is the recommended type of bed pan because of ease of use. A female urinal has proven useful during and after hospitalization because it lessens the need for sitting. It is imperative to avoid skin maceration under the cast. The patient will need instructions in adaptive techniques for bending and reaching and will need equipment to compensate for the loss of motion. A shoe lift may be needed.

Inability to flex the hip more than 25° makes sitting comfortably a challenge. Slouching in a chair to accommodate limited hip motion creates pressure on the back. Patients must have a custom foam cushion made that has a split seat with one half sloping to accommodate the fusion. Many companies and some foam stores will make custom seats. The Tall-Ette III arthro elevated toilet seat (Maddak Corporation, Pequannock, NJ) has one side sloped down to accommodate limited hip flexion. There are ergonomic office chairs with split adjustable seats as well as adjustable bicycle seats.

Resection Arthroplasty

A resection of the femoral head without use of an implant is called a girdlestone procedure or a resection arthroplasty. In the United States, this surgery is used primarily for patients with painful hips who are nonambulatory (e.g., patients with quadriplegia who have osteonecrosis or infection who are not candidates for a THA). Patients who develop an infection after a THA may have to have the implant removed, which leaves them with a resection arthroplasty until the infection can be irradiated with antibiotics (typically 6–10 weeks) and the prosthesis reimplanted. Physical therapy and occupational therapy are instrumental in helping the patient achieve some degree of independence between procedures. Sometimes patients are transferred to a skilled nursing facility when taking antibiotics because they are not capable of performing ADL at home because of other joint problems or lack of family support.

Resection arthroplasty results in a 5 to 9-cm shortening of the limb, and patients require a modified shoe sole extension. After a resection arthroplasty, most patients can manage only a touch-down gait because of the leg-length discrepancy and the inability of the muscle to support the hip. Pelvic motion helps to advance the leg during the swing phase. The lightest-weight material possible should be used for the shoe lift, which could be 2 to 3 in. in height. Exercise for motion is not emphasized after a resection arthroplasty, but assistive movements to the patient's tolerance are allowed. Isometrics are encouraged, as are knee and ankle exercises performed in the most comfortable position. Equipment and training in adaptive techniques are almost always needed after a resection arthroplasty because of difficulty in actively moving the hip and for patients with multiple joint involvement. It is important that patients have a program to maintain strength and functioning of other involved joints.

Conclusion

As in so many other areas of rehabilitation, research is needed to substantiate pre- and postoperative interventions (Munin, Kwoh, Glynn, Crosset, & Rushash, 1995). This task has been made easier with advancements in outcome instrumentation. The U.S. health care system is changing, and this is a perfect opportunity for all disciplines to combine efforts in patient education, development of practice standards, and collection of data.

References

Ayers, D. C., Evarts, C. M., & Parkinson, J. R. (1986). The prevention of heterotopic ossification in high-risk patients by low-dose radiation therapy after total hip arthroplasty. *Journal of Bone and Joint Surgery, 68A,* 1423–1430.

Beisaw, N. E., Comerota, A. J., & Groth, H. E. (1988). Dihydroergotamine heparin in the prevention of deep vein thrombosis after total hip arthroplasty. *Journal of Bone and Joint Surgery, 79B,* 2–9.

Bellamy, N., Buchanan, W. W., Goldsmith, C. H., Campbell, J., & Still, L. W. (1988). Validation study of the WOMAC: A health status instrument for measuring clinically important patient relevant outcomes to antirheumatic drug therapy in patients with osteoarthritis of the hip or knee. *Journal of Rheumatology, 15,* 1833–1844.

Berg, M., Bergman, B. R., & Hoborn, J. (1991). Ultraviolet radiation compared to an ultra-clean air enclosure: A comparison of air bacteria counts in operating rooms. *Journal of Bone and Joint Surgery, 73A,* 811–816.

Berg-Perier, M., Cederblad, A., & Persson, U. (1992). Ultraviolet radiation and ultra-clean air enclosures in operating rooms. *Journal of Arthroplasty, 7,* 457–463.

Berquist, D., Efsing, H. O., Hallbook, T., & Hedlund, T. (1979). Thromboembolism after elective and post-traumatic hip surgery: A controlled prophylactic trial with Dextran 70 and low dose heparin. *Acta Chirurgica Scandinavica, 145,* 213.

Bochner, R. M., Pellicci, P. M., & Lyden, J. P. (1988). Bipolar hemiarthroplasty for fracture of the femoral neck. *Journal of Bone and Joint Surgery, 70A,* 1001–1010.

Brand, R. A., Crowninshield, R. D., & Wittstock, C. E. (1982). A model of lower extremity muscular anatomy. *Journal of Biomechanical Engineering, 104,* 304–310.

Brander, V. A., Stulber, D., & Chang, R. Q. (1993). Life after total hip arthroplasty. *Bulletin on the Rheumatic Disease, 42,* 1–6.

Brandt, K., & Mankin, H. J. (1993). Pathogenesis of osteoarthritis. In W. M. Kelley, E. D. Harris, C. B. Sledge, & S. Ruddy (Eds.), *Textbook of rheumatology* (4th ed., pp. 1355–1393). Philadelphia: Saunders.

Brien, W. W., Warwick, B. J., Salvati, E. A., Wilson, P. D., & Pellicci, P. M. (1990). Acetabular reconstruction with a bipolar prosthesis and morseled bone grafts. *Journal of Bone and Joint Surgery, 72A,* 1230–1235.

Brower, A. C. (1994). Rheumatoid arthritis imaging. In J. H. Klippel & P. A. Dieppe (Eds.), *Rheumatology* (pp. 3.6.1–3.6.8). St Louis, MO: Mosby.

Burke, D. W., Gates, E. I., & Harris, W. H. (1984). Centrifugation as a method of improving tensile and fatigue properties of acrylic bone cement. *Journal of Bone and Joint Surgery, 66A,* 1265–1273.

Calandriello, B., & Grassi, G. (1982). Idiopathic osteonecrosis of the femoral head: Epidemiological and aetiological factors. *Italian Journal of Orthopaedic Trauma, 8* (Suppl.), 9–18.

Carnesale, P. G., Stewart, M. J., & Barnes, S. N. (1975). Acetabular disruption and central fracture-dislocation of the hip: A long-term study. *Journal of Bone and Joint Surgery, 57A,* 1054–1060.

Charnley, J. (1961). Arthroplasty of the hip: A new operation. *Lancet, 1,* 1129–1131.

Charnley, J. (1972). The long-term results of low-friction arthroplasty in the hip performed as a primary intervention. *Journal of Bone and Joint Surgery, 54A,* 61–69.

Enlow, L. G., Shields, R. K., Smith, K., Leo, K., & Miller, B. (1996). Total hip and knee replacement treatment programs: A report using consensus. *Journal of Sports Physical Therapy, 23,* 1–31.

Erickson, B., & Perkins, M. (1994). Interdisciplinary team approach in the rehabilitation of hip and knee arthroplasties. *American Journal of Occupational Therapy, 48,* 439–441.

Evarts, C. M., & Feil, E. J. (1971). Prevention of thromboembolic disease after elective surgery of the hip. *Journal of Bone and Joint Surgery, 53A*, 1271–1277.

Fisher, D. E. (1978). The role of fat embolism in the etiology of corticosteroid-induced avascular necrosis. *Clinical Orthopaedics and Related Research, 130*, 68–80.

Fisher, D. E., & Bickel, W. H. (1971). Corticosteroid-induced avascular necrosis. Journal of Bone and Joint Surgery, *53A,* 859–873.

Fitzgerald, R. H., Nolan, D. R., & Ilstrup, D. M. (1977). Deep wounds sepsis following total hip arthroplasty. *Journal of Bone and Joint Surgery, 59A*, 847.

Ganz, R., Klaue, K., Vinh, T. S., & Mast, J. W. (1988). A new periacetabular osteotomy for the treatment of hip dysplasias. *Clinical Orthopaedics and Related Research, 232*, 26–36.

Ganz, S. B., & Viellion, G. (1996). Pre and post surgical management of the hip and knee. In S. T. Wegener, B. L. Belza, & E. P. Gall (Eds.), *Clinical care in the rheumatic diseases*. Atlanta, GA: American College of Rheumatology.

Givens-Heiss, D. L., Krebs, D. E., Riley, P. O., Strickland, E. M., Fares, M., Hodge, W. A., & Mann, R. W. (1992). In vivo acetabular pressures during rehabilitation. Part II: Post-acute phase. *Physical Therapy, 72*, 700–705.

Goldenberg, D. (1993). Infectious arthritis. In H. R. Schumacher (Ed.), *The primer on the rheumatic diseases* (pp. 192–197). Atlanta, GA: Arthritis Foundation.

Gruebel-Lee, D. M. (1983). Anatomy of the hip joint. In D. M. Gruebel-Lee (Ed.), *Disorders of the hip* (pp. 1–24). Philadelphia: Lippincott.

Hammer, M., & Campy, J. (1993). *Reengineering the corporation*. New York: Harper Business.

Hanssen, A. D., Osmon, D. R., & Nelson, C. (1996). Prevention of deep periprosthetic joint infection. *Journal of Bone and Joint Surgery, 78A,* 458–471.

Harris, W. H., & McGann, W. A. (1986). Loosening of the femoral component after use of the medullary plug cementing technique. *Journal of Bone and Joint Surgery, 68A,* 1064–1066.

Harris, W. H., Salzman, E. W., Athanasoulis, C., & Waltman, A. C. (1977). Aspirin prophylaxis of venous thrombosis after total hip replacement. *New England Journal of Medicine, 297*, 1246–1252.

Hochberg, M. C., Altman, R. D., Brandt, K. D., Clark, B. C., Dieppe, P. A., Griffin, M. R., Moskowitz, R. Q., & Schnitzer, T. J. (1995). Guidelines for the medical management of osteoarthritis. Part I: Osteoarthritis of the hip. *Arthritis and Rheumatism, 38*, 1535–1540.

Johnson, M., Carmichael, J. E. H., Almond, H. G. A., & Loynes, R. P. (1978). Deep vein thrombosis following Charnley arthroplasty. *Clinical Orthopaedics and Related Research, 132*, 24–29.

Kaempffe, F. A., Lifeso, R. M., & Meinking, C. (1991). Intermittent pneumatic compression vs. coumadin: Prevention of deep vein thrombosis in the lower-extremity total joint arthroplasty. *Clinical Orthopaedics and Related Research, 269*, 89–97.

Klaue, K., Durnin, C. W., & Ganz, R. (1991). The acetabular rim syndrome: A clinical presentation of dysplasia of the hip. *Journal of Bone and Joint Surgery, 73B*, 423–429.

Krebs, D. E., Elbaum, L., Riley, P. O., Hodge, W. A., & Mann, R. W. (1991). Exercise and gait effects on in vivo hip contact pressures. *Physical Therapy, 71*, 301–309.

Lachiewicz, P. F., & Desman, S. M. (1988). The bipolar endoprosthesis in avascular necrosis of the femoral head. *Journal of Arthroplasty, 3*, 131–136.

Maderazo, E. R. G., Judson, S., & Pasternak, H. (1988). Late infections of total joint prothesis: A review and recommendation for prevention. *Clinical Orthopaedics and Related Research, 229*, 131–142.

Marvin, E. (1993). Osteonecrosis. In W. M. Kelley, E. D. Harris, C. B. Sledge, & S. Ruddy (Eds.), *Textbook of rheumatology* (4th ed., pp. 1628–1650). Philadelphia: Saunders.

Mattingly, D. A., Hopson, C. N., Kahn, A., & Giannestras, N. J. (1985). Aseptic loosening in metal-backed acetabular components for total hip replacement: A minimum five-year follow-up. *Journal of Bone and Joint Surgery, 67A,* 387–394.

Mattson, E., Bronstrom, L., & Linnarsson, D. (1990). Walking efficiency after cemented and uncemented total hip arthroplasty. *Clinical Orthopedics and Related Research, 254,* 170–179.

Mazieres, B. (1994). Osteonecrosis. In J. H. Klippel & P. A. Dieppe (Eds.), *Rheumatology* (pp. 7-41.1–7-41.8). St Louis, MO: Mosby.

McLeish, R. D., & Charnley, J. (1970). Abduction forces in the one legged stance. *Journal of Biomechanics, 3,* 191–209.

McGory, B. J., Stuart, M. J., & Sim, F. H. (1995). Participating in sports after hip and knee arthroplasty: Review of literature and survey of surgeon preference. *Mayo Clinic Proceedings, 70,* 342–348.

Melvin, J. L. (1989). *Rheumatic diseases in the adult and child: Occupational therapy and rehabilitation* (3rd ed.). Philadelphia: F. A. Davis.

Millis, M. B., Murphy, S. B., & Poss, R. (1995). Osteotomies about the hip for the prevention and treatment of osteoarthritis. *Journal of Bone and Joint Surgery, 77A,* 626–647.

Mueller, M. E., Sledge, C. B., & Poss, R. (1990). Report of the SICOT presidential commission on documentation and evaluation. *International Orthopaedics, 14,* 221–229.

Munin, M. C., Kwoh, C. K., Glynn, N., Crosset, L., & Rushash, H. E. (1995). Predicting discharge outcome after elective hip and knee arthroplasty. *American Journal of Physical Medicine and Rehabilitation, 74,* 294–301.

National Institute for Occupational Safety and Health. (1972). *Criteria for a recommended standard: Occupational exposure to ultraviolet radiation*. Washington, DC: U. S. Department of Health, Education, and Welfare.

National Institutes of Health. (1994). Consensus Development Conference on Total Hip Replacement, Bethesda, MD.

Neumann, D. A. (1996). Hip abductor muscle activity in persons with a hip prothesis while carrying loads in one hand. *Physical Therapy, 76,* 1320–1330.

Paiement, G. D., Schutzer, S. F., Wessinger, S. J., & Harris, W. H. (1992). Influence of prophylaxis on proximal venous thrombus formation after total hip arthroplasty. *Journal of Arthroplasty, 7,* 471–475.

Pellicci, P. M., Salvati, E. A., & Robinson, H. L. (1979). Mechanical failure of total hip arthroplasty requiring revision. *Journal of Bone and Joint Surgery, 61A,* 28–36.

Pennal, G. F., Davidson, J., Garside, H., & Plewes, J. (1980). Results of treatment of acetabular fractures. *Clinical Orthopaedics and Related Research, 151,* 115–123.

Perlau, R., Wilson, M. G., & Poss, R. (1996). Isolated proximal femoral osteotomy for treatment of residual congenital dysplasia or idiopathic osteoarthrosis of the hip: Five and ten year results. *Journal of Bone and Joint Surgery, 78A,* 1462–1467.

Phillips, T. W. (1987). The Bateman bipolar femoral head replacement: A fluoroscopic study of movement over a four year period. *Journal of Bone and Joint Surgery, 69A,* 761–764.

Platt, J. V., Hahn, R., Kessler, S., & McCarthy, D. Q. (1986). *Daily activities after your hip surgery.* Rockville, MD: American Occupational Therapy Association.

Poss, R., Brick, G., Wright, R. J., & Sledge, C. B. (1988). The effects of modern cement techniques on the longevity of total hip arthroplasty. *Orthopedic Clinics of North America, 19,* 591.

Poss, R., Robertson, D. D., & Walker, P. S. (1988). Anatomic stem design for press-fit and cemented application. In R. H. Fitzgerald Jr. (Ed.), *Non-cemented total hip arthroplasty* (pp. 343–363). New York: Raven Press.

Poss, R., & Sledge C. B. (1981). Surgery of the hip in rheumatoid arthritis. In W. N. Kelly, E. D. Harris, S. Ruddy, & C. B. Sledge (Eds.), *Textbook of rheumatology* (1st ed.). Philadelphia: Saunders.

Quinet, R. J., & Winter, E. G. (1992). Total joint replacement of the hip and knee. *Medical Clinics of North America, 76*, 1235–1251.

Radin, E. L., Ehrlich, M. G., & Chernack, R. (1978). Effect of repetitive impulsive loading on the knee joints of rabbits. *Clinical Orthopaedics and Related Research, 131*, 288–293.

Repo, R. V., & Finley, J. B. (1977). Survival of articular cartilage after controlled impact. *Journal of Bone and Joint Surgery, 59A*, 1068–1076.

Rimac, C. M., Wright, T. M., & McGill, D. L. (1986). The effect of centrifugation on the fracture properties of acrylic bone cement. *Journal of Bone and Joint Surgery, 68A*, 281–290.

Roberts, D. W., Poss, R., & Kelley, K. K. (1986). Radiographic comparison of cement techniques in total hip arthroplasty. *Journal of Arthroplasty, 1*, 241–247.

Rogers, P. W., Walsh, P. N., & Marden, V. H. (1978). Heparin and sulfinprazone to prevent venous thromboembolism after operations on the hip. *Journal of Bone and Joint Surgery, 60A*, 758–764.

Rohrle, H., Scholten, R., & Sigolotto, C. (1984). Joint forces in the human pelvis-leg skeleton during walking. *Journal of Biomechanics, 17*, 409–424.

Rothermal, J. E., Wessinger, J. B., & Stinchfield, F. E. (1973). Dextran 40 and thromboembolism in total hip replacement surgery. *Archives of Surgery, 106*, 135–143.

Rowe, C. R., & Lowell, J. D. (1961). Prognosis of fractures of the acetabulum. *Journal of Bone and Joint Surgery, 43A*, 30–38.

Rydell, N. (1966). Intra-vital measures of forces acting on the hip joint. In F. G. Evans (Ed.), *Studies on the anatomy and function of the bones and joints* (p. 52). New York: Springer-Verlag.

Schondorf, T. H., & Hey, D. (1976). Combined admithrombosis after hip joint surgery. *Haemostasis, 5*, 250–256.

Scott, R. D. (1984). Use of bipolar prosthesis and bone grafting in acetabular reconstruction. *Contemporary Orthopedics, 9*, 35–41.

Scott, R. D., Pomeroy, D., Oser, E., Schmidt, R., Turner, R., & Bierbaum, B. E. (1987). The results and technique of bipolar revision hip arthroplasty combined with acetabular grafting. *Orthopedic Transcripts, 11*, 450.

Shih, C. H., Du, Y. K., Lin, Y. H., & Wu, C. C. (1994). Muscular recovery around the hip joint after THA. *Clinical Orthopaedics and Related Research, 302*, 115–120.

Sledge, C. B. (1979). Correction of arthritic deformities in the lower extremity and spine. In D. J. McCarty (Ed.), *Arthritis and allied conditions* (pp. 563–588). Philadelphia: Lea & Febiger.

Smeltzer, S. C., & Bare, B. G. (1992). Brunner and Suddarth's textbook of medical-surgical nursing. Philadelphia: Lippincott.

Sponseller, P. D., McBeath, A. A., & Perpich, M. (1984). Hip arthrodesis in young patients: A long term follow-up study. *Journal of Bone and Joint Surgery, 66A*, 853–859.

Stewart, M. J., & Milford, L. W. (1954). Fracture-dislocation of the hip: An end result study. *Journal of Bone and Joint Surgery, 36A*, 315–322.

Strickland, E. M., Fares, M., Krebs, D. E., Riley, P. O., Given-Heiss, D. L., Hodge, W. A., & Mann, R. W. (1992). In vivo acetabular contact pressures during rehabilitation. Part I: Acute phase. *Physical Therapy, 72*, 691–699.

Sugioka, Y., Hotokebuchi, T., & Hideki, T. (1992). Transtrochanteric anterior rotational osteotomy for idiopathic and steroid induced necrosis of the femoral head. *Clinical Orthopaedics and Related Research, 277*, 111–120.

Sugioka, Y., & Ogata, K. (1991). Avascular necrosis of the femoral head. *Current Opinion in Othopedics, 2*, 437–441.

Trousdale, R. T., Ekkernkamp, A., & Ganz, R. (1995). Periacetabular and intertrochanteric osteotomy for the treatment of osteoarthrosis in dysplastic hips. *Journal of Bone and Joint Surgery, 77A*, 73–85.

Tsahakis, P. J., Brick, G. W., & Poss R. (1993). The hip. In W. M. Kelley, E. D. Harris, C. B. Sledge, & S. Ruddy (Eds.), *Textbook of rheumatology* (4th ed., pp. 1823–1833). Philadelphia: Saunders.

Upadhay, S. S., & Moulton, A. (1981). The long-term results of traumatic posterior dislocation of the hip. *Journal of Bone and Joint Surgery, 63A*, 548–551.

Upadhay, S. S., Moulton, A., & Srikrishnamurthy, K. (1983). An analysis of the late effects of traumatic posterior dislocation of the hip without fracture. *Journal of Bone and Joint Surgery, 65A*, 150–157.

Urist, M. R. (1948). Fracture-dislocation of the hip joint, the nature of the traumatic lesion, treatment, late complication and late results. *Journal of Bone and Joint Surgery, 30A*, 699–706.

Ware, J., & Sherbourne, C. (1992). The MOS 36 item short form health survey (SF-36). *Medical Care, 30*, 473–483.

Warner, J. P., Philip, J. H., Brodsky, G. L., & Thornhill, T. S. (1987). Studies of nontraumatic osteonecrosis. *Clinical Orthopaedics and Related Research, 225*, 104–127.

Wickiewicz, T. L., Roy, R. R., Powell, P. L., & Edgerton, V. R. (1983). Muscle architecture of the human lower limb. *Clinical Orthopaedics and Related Research, 179*, 275.

Wilson, M. G., Nikpoor, N., Aliabadi, P., Poss, R., & Weissman, B. N. (1989). The fate of acetabular allografts after bipolar revision arthroplasty of the hip: A radiographic review. *Journal of Bone and Joint Surgery, 71A*, 1469–1479.

Williams, J. F., & Svennsson, N. L. (1968). A force analysis of the hip joint. *Biomechanical Engineering, 3*, 365–370.

Wolf, L. R., Hozack, W. J., Balderston, R. A., Booth, R. E., & Rothman, R. H. (1992). Pulmonary embolism. *Journal of Arthroplasty, 74*, 465–469.

Zuckerman, J. D., Kummer, F. J., & Frankel, W. H. (1994). The effectiveness of a hospital based strategy to reduce the cost of total joint implants. *Journal of Bone and Joint Surgery, 76A*, 807–811.

Resources

Catalogs

Ali-Med, Inc.
297 High Street
Dedham, MA 02026-9135
800-225-2610

North Coast Medical, Inc.
187 Stauffer Boulevard
San Jose, CA 95125-1042
800-821-9319 or 408-283-1950

Sammons Preston, Inc.
P.O. Box 5071
Bolingbrook, IL 60440-5071
800-323-5547

Smith and Nephew, Inc.
One Quality Drive
P.O. Box 1005
Germantown, WI 53022-8205
800-545-7758

Textbook

Guide to independent living. (1988). Atlanta, GA: Arthritis Foundation (404-872-7100).

Internet

Abledata (www.abledata.com) is a database of more than 20,000 assistive devices and equipment including many items that are not in standard catalogs. Abledata has online support to help with specific searches. There is no fee.

Products

Tall-Ette III toilet seat
Maddak Corporation
6 Industrial Road
Pequannock, NJ 07440
(800-443-4926)

Theraband™
Hygenic Corporation
1245 Home Avenue
Akron, OH 44310
800-321-2135

Appendix 1
Postoperative Exercise Prescription for THA
Patient and Family Member Critical Pathway for THA

	After Your Surgery	POD 1	POD 2	POD 3–4	POD 4–5
Things you need to do	Cough and deep breathe every hour while awake Tell the nurse if you are uncomfortable at any time Assist the nurses in moving you in the bed	Continue coughing and deep breathing Ankle exercises every 2 hr Other exercises as instructed Ask questions about your positioning and hip precautions if you do not understand	Read a written list of exercises Ask questions about positioning and hip precautions if you do not understand	Watch videotapes on THA and coumadin Review booklet on coumadin Occupational therapy practitioner will discuss equipment needed for home	Review home safety, car transfers, and exercises with practitioner Review coumadin for after discharge with nurse Ask questions if you are unsure of anything
Treatment	You will be monitored by the nurse frequently Your tube from the incision will be checked along with your bandage Intravenous fluids and antibiotics will continue Wraps around both legs to promote circulation You will have a catheter to drain urine from your bladder	Skin pressure will be relieved by moving your position Your tube will be removed by the physician Suspension at night, out of suspension during the day with pillows between legs Wraps around both legs to promote circulation Catheter continues Compression cuffs on both legs	Intravenous line is removed Physician will change your bandage Continue with leg wraps A laxative will be given at bedtime if needed Catheter from bladder removed	Smaller bandage on hip or it will be left open to air Leg wraps discontinued on POD 4 Sling suspension at night should be discontinued	Equipment, prescriptions and follow-up appointments will be given
Diet	The nurses will check your abdomen and will let you know when you can start drinking fluids	Start on regular food	Regular diet	Regular diet	Regular diet
Activity	You will wake up in your bed in the recovery room Your operative leg will be supported by two slings You will remain in bed	Edge of bed for short periods You may get out of bed with a walker with the practitioner's help	Edge of bed or to chair with walker for meals Walk to bathroom with walker and with help	Perform exercises independently Increase distance walking Progress to crutches on POD 4	Walking greater than 50 ft. with crutches Stair training if needed
Discharge		Your expected length of stay and anticipated discharge destination will be reviewed with you If you are going to another facility for further rehabilitation, a call will be placed for the facility staff to come and visit you		Final destination on discharge will be confirmed You will be transported to a facility on POD 3 or 4, if planned	Discharge to home

Note: From Brigham and Women's Hospital, Boston, MA. Reprinted with permission.

Appendix 2
Multidisciplinary Documentation Total Hip Form

UNIVERSITY *of* PITTSBURGH
MEDICAL CENTER
St. Margaret

MULTIDISCIPLINARY DOCUMENTATION
TOTAL HIP DRG 209

I. Pre-Admission (initial at left if complete)

Nurse Practitioner to do H & P	Autologous Blood _____ #1 _____ #2 _____ #3
H & P PCP: Dr._____	Direct Donors _____ # units
EKG	Nursing Assessment Initiated
Urinalysis (Clean Catch Specimen)	Pre-op Instructions
CBC & DIFF	Video
PAC9 age 50 >	Review Surgical Procedure
Urine C&S if indicated	Pain Management Education
Social Service Card Sent	IS/C&DB Education
Anesthesia Consent	Unit Orientation
	Post-operative Instruction

Initials/Signature Section

II. Social/Home Status/Functional Status Pre-Admission

Home Status
☐ One Story
☐ Two Story
☐ Split Level
☐ Apartment
☐ PCBH
☐ ECF

Resides
☐ Alone
☐ Spouse
☐ Caretaker
☐ Family
   Members
☐ Other

Stairs
Outside #_____
☐ single ☐ double ☐ no rail
Inside #_____
☐ single ☐ double ☐ no rail
☐ No stairs/Doesn't use stairs

Occupation/Household Responsibilities/Comments:
☐ Cooking   ☐ Laundry
☐ Cleaning   ☐ Grocery Shopping

Comments: _____

Location of:
Bathroom ☐ 1st ☐ 2nd Floor
Bedroom   ☐ 1st ☐ 2nd Floor

Prior Community Services:
☐ Home Health   ☐ Access   ☐ Meals on Wheels
☐ Other _____

Ambulation
☐ Independent Without Device
☐ Independent With Device
_____
☐ Requires Assistance
☐ Non-Ambulatory
☐ Unknown

Transfers
☐ Independent
☐ Requires Assistance
☐ Total Dependence
☐ Unknown

Endurance
☐ Community Ambulator
☐ Household Ambulator
☐ N/A
☐ Unknown

Equipment Owned
☐ Standard/Wheeled/Platform Walker
☐ Straight/Quad Cane
☐ Wheelchair
☐ Axillary/Platform Crutches
☐ None/Unknown

Preliminary D/C Plans: Signature   Date

Physical Therapy Pre-op Evaluation

Comments: _____

Signature   Date

Occupational Therapy/ADL Pre-op Evaluation

Comments: _____

Signature   Date

NSG-470 (Rev. 6/94)

Appendix 2 (cont.)

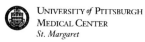

UNIVERSITY of PITTSBURGH
MEDICAL CENTER
St. Margaret

MULTIDISCIPLINARY DOCUMENTATION
TOTAL HIP DRG 209

DAY 1 DATE	Admission Day of Surgery			DAY 2 DATE	Post-op Day 1		
Medications	11-7	7-3	3-11	**Medications**	11-7	7-3	3-11
Pain Management Education				Pain Management Education			
Circle - Epidural, PCA, IM Injection				Circle - Epidural, PCA, IM Injection			
IV therapy per order				IV therapy per order			
Adequate Pain Relief				Adequate Pain Relief			
Prophylaxis/Medication Instruction				Prophylaxis/Medication Instruction			
				Blood transfusion if indicated			
				Nursing Assessment	11-7	7-3	3-11
				Alert & oriented x3			
Nursing Assessment	11-7	7-3	3-11	Neuro checks Q4° within normal limits			
Post-Op Nsg. Assess. form completed				Skin intact			
Alert & oriented x3				Hip Dsg. intact drainage may be present			
Neuro checks Q2° within normal limits				Drain intact			
Skin intact				Voiding s̄ problems via bedpan			
Hip Dsg. intact drainage may be present				Requiring intermittent catheterization			
Drain intact				Tolerating post-op lite or gen. diet			
Voiding s̄ problems via bedpan				Primary/Safety Standard of Care			
Requiring intermittent catheterization				**Respiratory Assessment**	11-7	7-3	3-11
Tolerating CL or post-op lite				Education Reinforced			
BS present				IS Q4° WA			
Primary/Safety Standard of Care				C & DB Q4°			
				O2_____ L as ordered			
				Respiration Unlabored			
				Activity	11-7	7-3	3-11
Respiratory Assessment	11-7	7-3	3-11	Abductor Pillow			
Respiratory Education				Begin Bed → Chair			
IS Q2° WA				Pulsatile stockings			
C & DB Q4°				TEDS when OOB			
O2_____ L as ordered				BSR Tx. if ordered			
Respirations Unlabored				Reinforce THR Education			

PT Signature_____
☐ 1x/day ☐ BID
TRANSFERS:
sup ≳ sit   ☐ **MOD** ☐ MAX ☐ MIN ☐ CS ☐Ⓢ ☐Ⓘ
sit ≳ stand ☐ **MOD** ☐ MAX ☐ MIN ☐ CS ☐Ⓢ ☐Ⓘ
AMBULATION: ☐ **MOD** ☐ MAX ☐ MIN ☐ CS ☐Ⓢ ☐Ⓘ
Device ☐ Walker ☐ Crutches ☐ Platform Walker
Distance _____ feet _____ WB status _____ ☐ WBAT ☐ PWB ☐ TDWB
HEP: ☐Ⓢ ☐Ⓘ QS, GS, AP, Heel Slides, Hip Abd.,SAQ x ≤ 10 reps
Pt. Education: ☐ Demonstrates understanding/observes precautions
_____
_____

Activity	11-7	7-3	3-11
Bedrest - turning side to side - Abd pillow			
Pulsatile stockings			
BSR Tx. if ordered			
THR Education			

Documentational Instructions

- Initial all applicable items

- (/) slash - indicates non-applicable items

- (V) variable - abnormal findings - must document in nurses notes

OT Signature_____
TRANSFERS:
Chair: ☐Ⓘ ☐Ⓘ c̄ device ☐ S ☐ MIN ☐ **MOD** ☐ MAX
Bed: supine ↔ sit   ☐Ⓘ ☐Ⓘ c̄ device ☐ S ☐ MIN ☐ MOD ☐ MAX
       sit ↔ stand ☐Ⓘ ☐Ⓘ c̄ device ☐ S ☐ MIN ☐ MOD ☐ MAX
LE ADL's:
    ☐ Review equipment
☐ UE screening (prn)
FIM SCALE ☐ Toilet   ☐ Tub/Shower   ☐ LE Bath   ☐ LE Drsg.
_____

Appendix 2 (cont.)

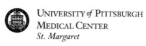

University *of* Pittsburgh
Medical Center
St. Margaret

MULTIDISCIPLINARY DOCUMENTATION
TOTAL HIP DRG 209

DAY 3 DATE	Post-op Day 2			**DAY 4** DATE	Post-op Day 3		
Medications	11 - 7	7 - 3	3 - 11	**Medications**	11 - 7	7 - 3	3 - 11
Pain Management Instruction Reinforced				Adequate Pain Relief			
Adequate Pain Relief				Heparin Lock			
Heparin Lock							
Prophylaxis/Medication Instruction				**Nursing Assessment**	11 - 7	7 - 3	3 - 11
Nursing Assessment	11 - 7	7 - 3	3 - 11	Neuro checks q8° within normal limits			
Alert & oriented x3				Skin intact			
Neuro checks Q8° within normal limits				Incision Care Instruction			
Skin intact				Dressing change			
Post-op Dsg. changed				Voiding s̄ problems in BR			
Drain intact				Check for BM/Document			
Voiding s̄ problems				DAT			
Check for BM & document on graphic				Primary/Safety Standard of Care			
Primary/Safety Standard of Care							
Respiratory Assessment	11 - 7	7 - 3	3 - 11	**Respiratory Assessment**	11 - 7	7 - 3	3 - 11
Education Reinforced				IS prn			
IS Q4° WA				Respirations unlabored			
C & DB Q4°							
O2 D/C				**Activity**	11 - 7	7 - 3	3 - 11
Respirations unlabored				Abductor pillow			
Activity	11 - 7	7 - 3	3 - 11	Ambulates to BR			
Abductor pillow				D/C Tx. if ordered			
Assist Amb. to BR / Walker				TEDS/Remove BID			
D/C Pulsatile stockings							
TEDS/Remove BID							
BSR Tx. if ordered							
Reinforce THR Education							

PT Signature_____
☐ Ambulatory devices to room
☐ 1x/day ☐BID
TRANSFERS:
  sup ⪦ sit ■ **MOD** ☐MAX ☐MIN ☐CS ☐Ⓢ ☐Ⓞ
  sit ⪦ stand ■ **MIN** ☐MAX ☐MOD ☐CS ☐Ⓢ ☐Ⓞ
AMBULATION: ■ **MOD** ☐MAX ☐MIN ☐CS ☐Ⓢ ☐Ⓞ
  Device ☐Walker ☐Crutches ☐Platform Walker
  Distance ☐≥ **25 feet** or _____ feet WB status ☐WBAT ☐PWB ☐TDWB
HEP: ☐Ⓞ ☐Ⓞ ≤ 10 reps

_____
_____
_____

OT Signature_____
TRANSFERS:
  Chair: ☐Ⓞ ☐Ⓞ c̄ device ☐S ■ **MIN** ☐MOD ☐MAX
  Bed: supine ↔ sit ☐Ⓞ ☐Ⓞ c̄ device ☐S ☐MIN ■ **MOD** ☐MAX
    sit ↔ stand ☐Ⓞ ☐Ⓞ c̄ device ☐S ☐MIN ■ **MOD** ☐MAX
  Toilet c̄ .equipment: ☐Ⓞ ☐Ⓞ c̄ device ☐S ■ **MIN** ☐MOD ☐MAX
  LE ADL's: ☐Ⓞ ☐Ⓞ c̄ device ☐S ■ **MIN** ☐MOD ☐MAX
☐Reinforce Education

_____
_____
_____

PT Signature_____
☐ 1x/day ☐BID
TRANSFERS:
  sup ⪦ sit ■ **MIN** ☐MAX ☐MOD ☐CS ☐Ⓢ ☐Ⓞ
  sit ⪦ stand ■ **CS** ☐MAX ☐MOD ☐MIN ☐Ⓢ ☐Ⓞ
AMBULATION: ■ **MIN** ☐MAX ☐MOD ☐CS ☐Ⓢ ☐Ⓞ
  Device ☐Walker ☐Crutches ☐Platform Walker
  Distance ☐≥ **50 feet** or _____ feet WB status ☐WBAT ☐PWB ☐TDWB
STAIRS: ■ **MOD** ☐MAX ☐MIN ☐CS ☐Ⓢ ☐Ⓞ
HEP: ☐Ⓞ ☐Ⓢ ≥ 10 reps
Family Education: ☐Ambulation ☐Transfers ☐Stairs ☐HEP ☐N/A

_____
_____
_____

OT Signature_____
TRANSFERS:
  Chair: ☐Ⓞ ☐Ⓞ c̄ device ☐S ■ **MIN** ☐MOD ☐MAX
  Bed: supine ↔ sit ☐Ⓞ ☐Ⓞ c̄ device ☐S ■ **MIN** ☐MOD ☐MAX
    sit ↔ stand ☐Ⓞ ☐Ⓞ c̄ device ☐S ■ **MIN** ☐MOD ☐MAX
  Toilet c̄ equipment: ☐Ⓞ ☐Ⓞ c̄ device ☐S ■ **MIN** ☐MOD ☐MAX
  LE ADL's: ☐Ⓞ ☐Ⓞ c̄ device ☐S ■ **MIN** ☐MOD ☐MAX
Assess Meal Prep (prn)

_____
_____
_____

Appendix 2 (cont.)

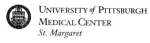

UNIVERSITY *of* PITTSBURGH
MEDICAL CENTER
St. Margaret

MULTIDISCIPLINARY DOCUMENTATION
TOTAL HIP DRG 209

DAY 5 DATE		Post-op Day 4			DAY 6 DATE		Post-op Day 5		
Medications		11-7	7-3	3-11	**Medications**	11-7	7-3	3-11	
Adequate Pain Relief					Adequate Pain Relief				
Nursing Assessment		11-7	7-3	3-11	**Nursing Assessment**	11-7	7-3	3-11	
Neuro checks q8° within normal limits					Neuro checks q8° within normal limits				
Skin intact					Skin intact				
Dressing change					Dressing change				
Voiding s̄ problems in BR					Voiding s̄ problem in BR				
Check for BM/Document					Elimination s̄ difficulty				
DAT					DAT				
Primary/Safety Standard of Care					Primary/Safety Standard of Care				
Activity		11-7	7-3	3-11	**Activity**	11-7	7-3	3-11	
Abductor pillow					Abductor pillow				
Amb. with Walker					Amb. with Walker				
TEDS/Remove BID					TEDS/Remove BID				

PT Signature_____
☐ 1x/day ☐ BID
TRANSFERS:
sup ≷ sit ☐① ☐MAX ☐MIN ☐MOD ☐CS ☐Ⓢ
sit ≷ stand ☐① ☐MAX ☐MIN ☐MOD ☐CS ☐Ⓢ
AMBULATION: ☐① ☐MAX ☐MIN ☐MOD ☐CS ☐Ⓢ
Device ☐ Walker ☐ Crutches ☐ Platform Walker
Distance ☐ ≥ 50 feet or _____ feet
STAIRS: ☐CS ☐MAX ☐MOD ☐MIN ☐Ⓢ ☐①
HEP: ☐① ☐Ⓢ ≥ 10 reps

_____
_____
_____

PT Signature_____
☐ 1x/day ☐ BID
TRANSFERS:
sup ≷ sit ☐① ☐MAX ☐MOD ☐MIN ☐CS ☐Ⓢ
sit ≷ stand ☐① ☐MAX ☐MOD ☐MIN ☐CS ☐Ⓢ
AMBULATION: ☐① ☐MAX ☐MOD ☐MIN ☐CS ☐Ⓢ
Device ☐ Walker ☐ Crutches ☐ Platform Walker
Distance ☐ ≥ 100 feet or _____ feet
STAIRS: ☐① ☐MAX ☐MOD ☐MIN ☐CS ☐Ⓢ
☐0 ☐1 ☐2 ☐Rails ☐Cane ☐Crutches ☐None
HEP: ☐① ☐Ⓢ
Education: ☐ Demonstrates understanding/observation of precautions

_____
_____
_____

OT Signature_____
TRANSFERS:
Chair: ☐① ☐①c̄ device ☐S ☐MIN ☐MOD ☐MAX
Bed: supine ↔ sit ☐① ☐①c̄ device ☐S ☐MIN ☐MOD ☐MAX
sit ↔ stand ☐① ☐①c̄ device ☐S ☐MIN ☐MOD ☐MAX
Toilet c̄ equipment: ☐① ☐①c̄ device ☐S ☐MIN ☐MOD ☐MAX
Tub/Shower: ☐① ☐①c̄ device ☐MIN ☐MOD ☐MAX
LE ADL's: ☐① ☐①c̄ device ☐S ☐MIN ☐MOD ☐MAX
Meal Prep (prn) ☐① ☐①c̄ device ☐S ☐MIN ☐MOD ☐MAX

_____
_____
_____

OT Signature_____
TRANSFERS:
Chair: ☐① ☐①c̄ device ☐S ☐MIN ☐MOD ☐MAX
Bed: supine ↔ sit ☐① ☐①c̄ device ☐S ☐MIN ☐MOD ☐MAX
sit ↔ stand ☐① ☐①c̄ device ☐S ☐MIN ☐MOD ☐MAX
Toilet c̄ equipment: ☐① ☐①c̄ device ☐S ☐MIN ☐MOD ☐MAX
Tub/Shower: ☐① ☐①c̄ device ☐S ☐MIN ☐MOD ☐MAX
LE ADL's: ☐① ☐①c̄ device ☐S ☐MIN ☐MOD ☐MAX
Meal Prep (prn) ☐① ☐①c̄ device ☐S ☐MIN ☐MOD ☐MAX

_____
_____
_____

Initials/Signature Section	**Initials/Signature Section**

Appendix 2 (cont.)

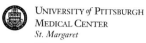

UNIVERSITY *of* PITTSBURGH
MEDICAL CENTER
St. Margaret

**MULTIDISCIPLINARY DOCUMENTATION
TOTAL HIP DRG 209**

Discharge Instructions

Occupational Therapy

Transfers

							ADL's						
Commode:	Ⓘ	Ⓘc̄ Devices	SUPV	MIN	MOD	MAX	Dressing:	Ⓘ	Ⓘc̄ Devices	SUPV	MIN	MOD	MAX
Bed ≥ Chair:	Ⓘ	Ⓘc̄ Devices	SUPV	MIN	MOD	MAX	Bath/Hygiene:	Ⓘ	Ⓘc̄ Devices	SUPV	MIN	MOD	MAX
Bath/Shower:	Ⓘ	Ⓘc̄ Devices	SUPV	MIN	MOD	MAX	Homemaking Meal Prep:	Ⓘ	Ⓘc̄ Devices	SUPV	MIN	MOD	MAX

Patient demonstrated ability to incorporate joint protection and safety into ADL's. ☐ Yes ☐ No

Comments: _____

_____

_____ Signature: _____

Physical Therapy

GOALS:

					Achieved	Not Achieved
☐	1. I SUPV CS MIN transfers supine < >sit				☐	☐
☐	2. I SUPV CS MIN transfers sit < > stand				☐	☐
☐	3. I SUPV CS MIN "stairs" ↑↓ with ☐ 0 ☐ 1 ☐ 2 rails and/or devices:				☐	☐
	Device: ☐ cane ☐ crutches ☐ platform crutch ☐ walker (↑↓ 1 step) ☐ other _____					
	☐ stairs not required					
☐	4. I SUPV CS MIN ambulation with device				☐	☐
	Device: ☐ cane ☐ crutches ☐ platform crutch ☐ platform walker ☐ walker ☐ other _____					
☐	5. Ambulation _____ feet or greater ☐ NWB ☐ TDWB ☐ PWB ☐ WBAT				☐	☐
☐	6. Ⓘ with written home exercise program				☐	☐
☐	7. Patient demonstrates understanding of precautions.				☐	☐
☐	8. _____				☐	☐
☐	9. _____				☐	☐
☐	10. _____				☐	☐

Other Physical Findings: _____

_____

_____

A: _____ out of _____ goals achieved. The following goals were not achieved 2° to: _____

_____

_____

Comments: _____

P: Pt D/C to: ☐ Home ☐ PCH ☐ ECF ☐ REHAB Facility ☐ Other _____

Follow-up:

Signature _____

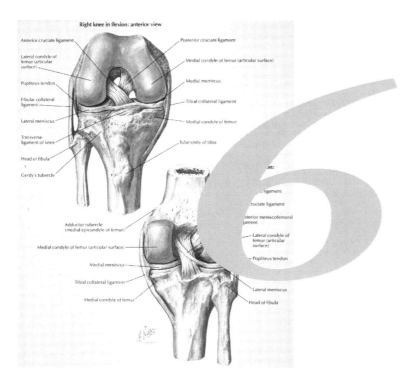

KNEE SURGERY AND REHABILITATION

Thomas Sculco, MD, Sandy B. Ganz, MS, PT, Jill Noaker, OTR, CHT, and Mary Ann Jacobs, RN

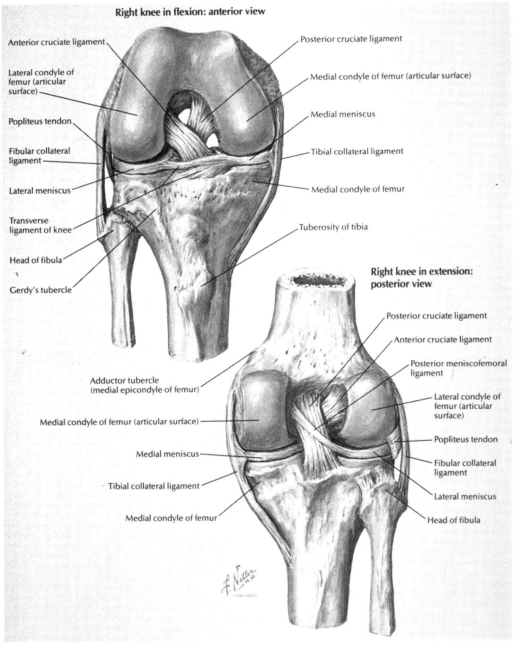

Right knee in flexion: anterior view

Anterior cruciate ligament

Lateral condyle of femur (articular surface)

Popliteus tendon

Fibular collateral ligament

Lateral meniscus

Transverse ligament of knee

Head of fibula

Gerdy's tubercle

Posterior cruciate ligament

Medial condyle of femur (articular surface)

Medial meniscus

Tibial collateral ligament

Medial condyle of femur

Tuberosity of tibia

Right knee in extension: posterior view

Adductor tubercle (medial epicondyle of femur)

Medial condyle of femur (articular surface)

Medial meniscus

Tibial collateral ligament

Medial condyle of femur

Posterior cruciate ligament

Anterior cruciate ligament

Posterior meniscofemoral ligament

Lateral condyle of femur (articular surface)

Popliteus tendon

Fibular collateral ligament

Lateral meniscus

Head of fibula

Anatomy of the knee in flexion (anterior) and extension (posterior). Copyright 1989. Novartis. Reprinted with permission from the *Atlas of Human Anatomy*, illustrated by Frank H. Netter, MD. All rights reserved.

Reconstructive surgery in the knee with arthritis has expanded tremendously during the past decade with technological advances in arthroscopy and joint replacement arthroplasty. Severe degenerative joint disease with complex knee deformity, associated bone deficits, and soft-tissue imbalances now can be reconstructed successfully with an array of modular knee implants that allow the surgeon to customize the prosthesis to the patient's problem. Procedures that were only possible through large open arthrotomies a few years ago are now performed routinely arthroscopically. Along with these technical advances, the pressures of managed care and day-surgery centers have encouraged a more rapid mobilization of patients and the associated need for more intense inpatient and ambulatory rehabilitation. The orthopedic surgeon, nursing staff members, and therapy staff members more than ever must work as a coordinated team with effective communication and common goals. Along with this close partnership, the practitioner must be able to evaluate and modify therapy programs by using basic knowledge of the surgical procedures and the goals of the reconstruction. This is possible only with an improved knowledge base. This chapter will deal with the decision-making process for selecting surgery, the array of procedures available, and the role of surgical rehabilitation. The rehabilitation section will discuss the specific methods for achieving these objectives.

Orthopedic Evaluation

The surgeon's first step in the orthopedic evaluation of a person with a painful knee is to develop a working diagnosis on the basis of the patient's history, radiographs, laboratory tests, and physical examination. This requires formulating appropriate questions regarding knee function that concern duration of symptoms, precipitating cause of pain, localization of pain, activities that exacerbate pain, and response to rest and medication. More specific questions about locking, buckling, swelling, crepitus, and stiffness are helpful.

The physical examination focuses on observation of the knee and its function and examination of knee motion and stability and the other joints in the affected lower extremity. An examination of the contralateral knee is important and may be used as a baseline for normal function in the patient if it is unaffected. The gait pattern is extremely important in determining function of the knee joint in a loaded and active mode. Functional evaluation and outcome measures are discussed in the section on total knee arthroplasty (TKA) on page 136 later in this chapter.

A patient with a painful knee who is a surgical candidate should have a basic radiograph as part of his or her initial evaluation. Knee radiographs (anteroposterior) should always be taken while bearing weight to determine actual joint configuration and cartilage narrowing. Lateral and patellar views should be routine. An anteroposterior (tunnel) view with the knee flexed may provide additional information about joint space narrowing, which may not be appreciated on a full-extension loaded view.

Magnetic resonance imaging (MRI) is indicated when the diagnosis indicates damage to the soft tissues about the knee joint. It is particularly useful in evaluating the menisci and ligamentous structures. Avascular necrosis of the distal femur or proximal tibia can be seen on an MRI before it is apparent on plain radiographs.

If inflammatory arthritis is suspected, serological studies (rheumatoid factor) and sedimentation rate may assist with making the diagnosis. If crystalline synovitis produced by gout or pseudogout (i.e., calcium pyrophosphate dihydrate deposition disease) is suspected, or if knee infection is a possibility, knee aspiration for crystalline evaluation and cultures should be performed.

Most knee disorders can be classified into categories. Table 1 categorizes disorders as inflammatory or mechanical. This simplifies all disorders that may affect the knee joint, and it provides a framework to help classify the nature of the knee dysfunction. A classification such as this helps in the therapeutic approach to the patient problem. Nonsteroidal anti-inflammatory drugs (NSAIDs) may be useful in disorders that are primarily inflammatory, but they will provide only little relief if there is a major mechanical component to the pathology.

Table 1. Classification of Knee Disorders

Inflammatory
- Synovium
  —RA, psoriatic arthritis, inflammatory arthritides
  —Hemorrhagic: posttraumatic, hemophilia, pigmented villonodular synovitis
  —Crystalline synovitis: gout, pseudogout
- Joint
  —Posttraumatic arthritis
  —Infection
  —OA with inflammation
- Tendon, ligament, bursa
  —Patellar tendon, hamstring tendons
  —Pes anserinus, prepatellar, infrapatellar bursitis
  —Posttraumatic tendon, ligament, or bursal inflammation

Mechanical
- Meniscus tear
- Loose body
- Joint incongruity (OA)
- Avascular necrosis (medial femoral condyle)
- Osteochondritis dissecans

Instability
- Cruciate ligament insufficiency
- Patellar subluxation

Medical and Rehabilitative Management

For most conditions affecting the knee joint, a conservative program is sufficient treatment. The basic goals of treatment are to control pain and inflammation with medication and then rehabilitate the knee joint. Guidelines for the medical management of osteoarthritis (OA), which is predominately a mechanical problem, were developed by the American College of Rheumatology (ACR) in 1995 (Hochberg et al., 1995) and are summarized in Table 2. Note that nonopioid analgesics (e.g., acetaminophen) are the recommended first agents to be used for this disease, not NSAIDs.

Anti-inflammatory medications are used for diseases such as rheumatoid arthritis (RA) and psoriatic arthritis. For severe inflammatory OA of the knee, a short 7 to 10-day course of anti-inflammatory medications may be used.

NSAIDs may be poorly tolerated in older patients and those with a history of gastritis or ulcer disease. NSAIDs inhibit prostaglandin synthesis, which then decreases mucus and bicarbonate secretions, thus drastically decreasing the gastrointestinal mucosal defense factors. This may lead to ulcerations of the mucosal lining (Ward & Jackson, 1992). Misoprosol is the drug of choice in the prevention of NSAID-induced gastric and duodenal ulcers. Some NSAIDs, particularly indomethacin, may cause dizziness and headaches. Renal and hepatic complications from NSAIDs are rare but may be catastrophic. There are a series of new anti-inflammatory medications that will be available

Table 2. American College of Rheumatology Guidelines for Management of the Patient With OA of the Knee

---

Nonpharmacological therapy
- Patient education
  - —Self-management programs (arthritis self-help course)
  - —Health professional social support via telephone contact
- Weight loss (if overweight)
- Physical therapy
  - —ROM exercises
  - —Quadriceps-strengthening exercises
  - —Assistive devices for ambulation
- Occupational therapy
  - —Joint protection and energy conservation
  - —Assistive devices for ADL
- Aerobic exercise program

Pharmacological therapy
- Nonopioid analgesics (acetaminophen)
- Intra-articular steroid injections
- Topical analgesics (capsaicin, methylsalicylate creams)
- Nonsteroidal anti-inflammatory drugs
- Opioid analgesics (propoxyphene, codeine, oxycodone)

Note. From "Guidelines for the medical management of osteoarthritis," by M. C. Hochberg, R. D. Altman, K. D. Brandt, B. M. Clark, P. A. Dieppe, M. R. Griffin, R. W. Moskowitz, and T. J. Schnitzer, 1995, *Arthritis and Rheumatism*, 38, pp. 1541–1546. Copyright 1995 by the American College of Rheumatology and Lippincott-Raven Publishers. Reprinted with permission.

in the next few years called COX-2 (cyclooxygenase-2) selective inhibitors that may be effective agents without causing gastrointestinal disruption.

When knee synovitis is acute and not responsive to anti-inflammatory medication, an intra-articular injection of cortisone is often used. For soft-tissue inflammatory problems, cortisone may be injected around or into tendon, bursa, and rarely ligamentous areas. Too frequent a repetition of cortisone injections should not be performed because damage may occur in tendon and ligamentous structures. Generally, it is recommended that no more than three cortisone injections be given per year.

Nonpharmacological treatments for OA are emphasized in the ACR guidelines. Patient education and exercise are essential. Therapeutic exercise should be prescribed routinely for patients with any dysfunction of the knee. The quadriceps and hamstring muscles rapidly weaken with a painful knee as off-loading (reduced weight bearing) of the affected limb occurs. Exercise programs should be isometric to start and progress to more vigorous resistance exercises, depending on degree of pain and inflammation and the patient's lifestyle. Aerobic programs in water, walking, or on available equipment can be used as symptoms lessen. For more chronic knee disorders, individual programs should be developed for the patient to maintain strength, function, and range of motion (ROM) (Minor, 1998).

Joint protection through avoidance of provocative activities that aggravate the underlying knee condition is basic to recovery. Persistence of heavy aerobic or running programs can greatly increase knee pain and retard recovery. An inflammatory problem may become more mechanical and chronic from continued abuse of the knee joint by stressful activities. Recreational exercises and activities may be pursued but not to the extent that pain is increased.

External splinting with passive constraints such as knee braces provides some improved function in patients with mild inflammatory or mechanical problems. Bracing can compensate for major instability of the knee, but it must severely restrict motion and function to truly stabilize. The more constraining braces tend to be cumbersome and not well tolerated. Knee braces without restraints tend to improve the proprioceptive feedback for patients, thus making them more conscious of being protective of the knee during activities that might lead to worsening of knee pain. Cryotherapy with ice or cooling devices tends to be more effective for inflammation than warm compresses, which can increase local swelling and exacerbate the underlying condition. Surgical intervention is indicated for the patient with an unremitting mechanical or inflammatory condition. Various procedures are available, depending on the disorder.

Disease Progression in the Knee

Arthritic conditions of the knee joint by their definition imply joint destruction. More precisely, hyaline (articular) cartilage undergoes degradation with fissuring, fibrillation, and complete degeneration of its substance and is a result of a combination of biochemical and mechanical stimuli. It may be provoked by several causes:

- trauma to the joint surfaces with damage to the articular surface
- overload to the cartilage surfaces accompanying meniscus or ligamentous injury

- infection, or
- (in the case of inflammatory arthritides such as RA) by synovitis that releases destructive enzymes.

Regardless of the inciting cause, the end result is the same—articular cartilage damage, usually focal in the case of OA and more global in RA and psoriatic arthritis. Arthritis additionally causes secondary damage to the supporting soft tissues. Soft-tissue stabilizers of the knee joint, particularly the collateral ligaments, become shortened on the involved side of the arthritic knee, thus resulting in deformity and malalignment from loss on the condylar surface of the joint. The soft-tissue symmetry must be balanced at the time of arthroplasty, and bone loss, if severe, may require bone grafting.

OA

OA tends to be localized to a single compartment, most commonly medial, but the patellofemoral compartment is often damaged when the tibiofemoral compartment is abnormal. In the knee joint, 60% of the load is transmitted normally through the medial compartment; therefore, it tends to be damaged more frequently. Furthermore, when the medial compartment articular cartilage narrows, the knee tends to drift into a varus (bowed) position, and this further increases the transfer of load to the medial joint and accelerates the articular destruction on the medial joint surfaces. The soft tissues become contracted on the medial side of the joint as the medial compartment narrows, and the lateral soft tissues and ligamentous complex become lax.

In the case of lateral compartment arthritis, the joint space narrows laterally, and the knee tends to drift into a more valgus deformity ("knock-knee"). This is associated with contracture of the lateral ligamentous structures and medial laxity. There may be associated flexion and rotational deformities with both varus and valgus malalignment that produce further complex soft-tissue imbalances. In the knee with OA, bone proliferates (osteophytosis) in a futile attempt to resurface the joint, and these osteophytes or spurs may severely limit joint motion and produce great pain as the capsule and soft tissues rub over these rough and irregular surfaces (Figure 1). Malalignment commonly occurs when there is unicompartmental damage in the knee joint. In the most severe cases, this may accelerate the tendency for transverse subluxation of the joint. It is paramount in prosthetic reconstruction of a joint with OA that the tightened and contracted soft tissues be lengthened during surgery so that they are symmetrical with the lax side of the joint. The implant then tends to symmetrically balance the joint as the deformity is corrected.

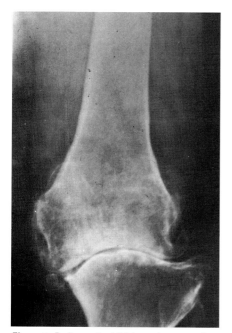

Figure 1. Radiograph of OA knee demonstrating focal joint destruction with osteophyte (spur) formation.

Inflammatory Arthritis

Inflammatory arthritis tends to affect the knee joint more globally as the destructive lyosomal enzymes, collagenoses, and cytokines are released throughout the knee joint

(Figure 2). The synovium in these patients tends to be hypertrophic and the joint quite swollen. In the most severe instances, pannus (a combination of synovial and granulation tissue) may directly invade subchondral and cartilage surfaces. Not only is hyaline cartilage destroyed in this inflammatory process, but the menisci and cruciate and collateral ligaments are often severely damaged. Laxity is more of a problem than stiffness in RA or inflammatory knee arthritis. Osteophytes tend to be infrequent in the rheumatoid knee, unless the disease has progressed to a quiescent phase and the joint has become secondarily destroyed by increased mechanical loads. In these cases, the joint may look similar to that in OA.

In both OA and inflammatory arthritis, as the joint destruction progresses, the underlying subchondral bone will tend to collapse; this produces defects within the joint surfaces. In RA, there is often osteopenia from the disease itself and from corticosteroid medications that can further accelerate bony collapse.

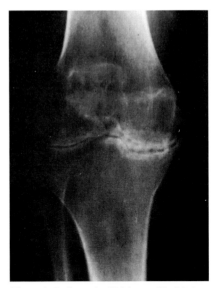

Figure 2. Radiograph of RA knee with global joint space narrowing, osteopenia, and absence of osteophytes.

Surgical Options

On the basis of the pathological findings in the arthritic joint, a series of surgical procedures are available when nonsurgical measures are not sufficient. These surgical interventions fall into five categories: (a) arthroscopy, (b) synovectomy, (c) chondrocyte implantation, (d) osteotomy, and (e) total knee arthroplasty. The following section will discuss the range of procedures available for alleviating pain and increasing function in the knee joint with arthritis. Indications, outcomes, and limitations will be presented.

Arthroscopy

Debridement procedures. Debridement procedures are performed arthroscopically and are most beneficial if there is a mechanical component to the patient's knee symptoms. A degenerated torn meniscus is commonly encountered in knee arthritis and may produce symptoms of intermittent locking and swelling. An MRI is helpful in confirming the diagnosis of a torn meniscus preoperatively, but many patients with an arthritic knee will have meniscal damage. In arthroscopic debridement, the degenerative and torn meniscal fragment is removed, and the knee is lavaged to remove debris. This smoothing and shaving subtotal meniscectomy will reduce the locking and mechanical symptoms, but chondroplasty of the arthritic surfaces has not been demonstrated to provide long-term relief. In fact, excessive debridement of arthritic surfaces may expose subchondral bone and accelerate the breakdown of hyaline cartilage (McLaren, Blokker, Fowler, Roth, & Rock, 1991; Novak & Bach, 1993; Rand, 1991).

During arthroscopic surgery, copious amounts of irrigating fluid are lavaged through the knee joint. This can amount to 10–12 L of fluid for procedures that are an hour in duration. It is this lavage effect that clears the joint of inflammatory cells and joint debris, and it may in fact provide much of the relief seen with arthroscopic surgery of the arthritic knee (Gibson, White, Chapman, & Strachan, 1992). This is particularly true in patients who have pseudogout (i.e., a crystalline synovitis with deposition of calcium pyrophosphate) or gout (i.e., uric acid crystals in the hyaline and meniscal cartilage). These crystalline materials are extremely irritating to the synovial lining and lead to major joint effusions. Benefit from the irrigation of these crystals and other debris from the joint is usually self-limited with amelioration of joint symptoms and lasts for only a 3 to 6-month period. Arthroscopic surgery is performed in an ambulatory day-surgery environment, and simple lavage may be carried out in an office setting by either an orthopedic surgeon or a rheumatologist.

Arthroscopic Rehabilitation

Rehabilitation of patients after arthroscopic surgery for debridement or for removal of a torn meniscal fragment tends to be quite rapid. The procedure is performed in a day-surgery setting with discharge several hours after recovery from anesthesia. Regional and (in some cases) local anesthesia can be used for arthroscopic surgery. Cryotherapy is instituted immediately after surgery and, when available, a Cryocuff™ device (Aircast, Inc., Summit, NJ) is recommended instead of ice packs because of its circumferential and compressive properties. Patients are discharged with crutches or a cane for protected or partial weight bearing, but these aids are usually discontinued several days after an uncomplicated arthroscopic procedure.

ROM exercises and strengthening exercises of the knee are begun the day after the procedure. Motion usually returns without difficulty. In procedures requiring extensive debridement, recovery may be more prolonged, protected weight bearing is continued for a longer period, and exercise progress is gradual. If the gait training and home instruction are given at a preoperative visit and not by a practitioner after the procedure, then the staff members of the day-surgery unit should be competent in assisting the patient with the ambulatory device and in answering questions.

Because the procedure is usually performed through three 1/4 to 1/2-in. portals, only one suture is needed to close each incision; these are removed 7 to 10 days after surgery. Outpatient physical therapy, if needed, will begin at this time. The program must balance muscle strengthening with flexibility exercises while protecting healing tissue from overload. Overzealous therapy, although avoiding the deleterious effects of immobility and disuse, can increase swelling and may cause a patella femoral syndrome, which is an irritation of the patella cartilage from poor tracking over the femur caused by joint swelling and weakness of the quadriceps muscles. As the wound heals, the patient progresses to a more vigorous program developed on the basis of available equipment and functional goals.

Open and closed kinetic chain exercises (or both) improve motion and strength. The concept of the kinetic chain permits one to view the action of the lower extremity as a functional unit. Open-chain exercises have the foot off the ground during exercise—sitting and flexing and extending the knee. Closed-chain exercises are performed when the foot is in contact with a supporting surface—the ground or a pedal. Closed-chain exercises appropriate to the patient's postoperative status are considered more functional and safer for the patella femoral joint (Steindler, 1955; Yack, Collins, & Wheldon, 1993). The effective treatment of musculoskeletal knee pain and dysfunction requires a broad knowledge of modalities and gait-training exercise principles.

Crutches or a cane should be used until the incision is healed and the antalgic nature of the gait has ceased. Discontinuation of aids too early may be detrimental because walking with a limp is fatiguing and can increase swelling. A cane should be used if motion or strength is limited. Swelling may persist for weeks, and ice applications are recommended, particularly after exercise. If a flexion contracture persists, passive stretching and prone lying are recommended (1 to 2 times a day for 30-min sessions).

Arthroscopic menisectomy for an uncomplicated torn meniscus or removal of a loose body generally produces excellent results with rapid recovery and elimination of mechanical symptoms. Results tend to be less predictable in the patient with OA for whom there may be a persistence of joint pain as a result of the chronic nature of the disease.

Synovectomy

Arthroscopic synovectomy is the procedure for intractable hypertrophic synovitis that is unresponsive to medical management (Ogilvie-Harris & Weisleder, 1995; Ogilvie-Harris & Fitsialos, 1991). Besides RA and PA, this procedure is an effective intervention for hemophilic arthropathy and synovial proliferation disorders such as pigmented villonodular synovitis (Huo & Galloway, 1994; Schumacher, 1993). This rare disease is a slowly progressive benign proliferation of synovial tissue, but the synovial hypertrophy tends to be quite invasive and may penetrate into the ligamentous and meniscal surfaces (Convery, Lyon, & Laverna 1994; Figure 3).

Arthroscopic synovectomy requires removal of synovial tissue from all compartments of the knee and, therefore, tends to be a far more extensive procedure than arthroscopic menisectomy. The synovial tissue may be quite vascular, which leads to bleeding from the surfaces, and a large hemarthrosis may occur after synovectomy. A drain may be used in these patients for 6 to 8 hr. Recovery is slower because of the extensive nature of the surgery. Recurrent synovitis does occur in these patients, but it could take years to develop. Patients experience marked improvement of their knee pain after arthroscopic synovectomy because of the reduction in knee synovial tissue and reduction in the accompanying severe joint effusions.

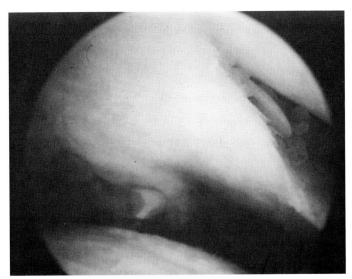

Figure 3. Photograph of arthroscopic synovectomy of rheumatoid knee demonstrating synovitis involving joint and meniscus.

A synovectomy by arthrotomy is less frequent because of the advances in arthroscopic technique and because of the lengthier recovery time. In RA, pain relief is excellent; however, the procedure does not halt the progression of the disease (Ishikawa, Ohno, & Hirohata, 1986).

Rehabilitation for an open synovectomy (arthrotomy) usually follows the guidelines of a TKA described later in this chapter. Synovectomy is often more painful than a TKA, so the epidural catheter may remain in place for a day longer. Transfer to a rehabilitation facility usually is not necessary, but home therapy is common.

For pigmented villonodular synovitis, an anteroposterior incision is often needed for meticulous excision of synovial tissue. The tendency toward flexion contracture is increased because of the pain with stretching the posterior incision during extension. Again, the rehabilitation program follows that of a TKA but with greater attention to skin care and positioning.

Radiation Synovectomy

Radiation synovectomy evolved as an alternative to surgical synovectomy. With the advent of arthroscopy synovectomy and more effective medications for inflammatory rheumatic diseases, this procedure has become uncommon in the United States. It is difficult to obtain the radiochemicals in the United States, but the procedure continues to be used in Europe and in other parts of the world.

Radiation synovectomy is the removal of the inflamed synovial tissue by radiochemical ablation of the synovial lining via intra-articular injection of a radionuclide (90-yttrium) attached to a carrier particle. The carrier particle is phagocytosed by the synovial cells, and the radioactivity provokes their cell death as well as the death of surrounding cells to a depth consistent with the capabilities of the radionuclide. The dose to the joint space is high (5,000–10,000 rad), but the whole-body dose is limited because 90-yttrium, a beta-emitting radionuclide, has a tissue penetration of less than 12 mm (Deutsch, Brodack, & Deutsch, 1993).

Numerous studies in Europe have documented the effectiveness of radiation synovectomy in treating RA with 60% to 80% good to excellent results. In a review of 29 articles describing the results of radiation synovectomy for RA, there were reports of 1,681 knees with 66% good to excellent results (Deutsch et al., 1993). Many of these studies treated all stages of the disease. The treatment is most effective in patients with little or no joint damage (i.e., radiographic Stage I or early Stage II). If radiation synovectomy is performed within these parameters, the beneficial effects are equivalent to that of surgical synovectomy, which is 3 to 5 years (Laurin, Desmarchais, Daziano, Gariepy, & Derome, 1974).

Leakage of the radioactivity from the joint space is the main concern, which has been reported to occur in 10% to 25% of the injected doses, and there are effects on nontarget organs (Dunscombe, Bhattacharyya, & Dale, 1976; Dunscombe & Ramsey, 1980). Although the agent is still currently in use in Europe, and no long-term adverse effects have been reported, researchers in the United States have been investigating potential agents that might reduce the burden to nontarget organs and still be as effective as 90-yttrium. Clinical trials with 165 dysprosium-ferric hydroxide macroaggregate have demonstrated its effectiveness in the treatment of early-stage RA as well as other inflammatory joint diseases. A good to excellent result was noted in approximately

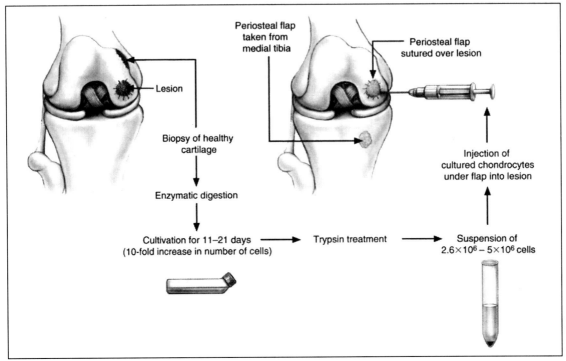

Figure 4. From "Treatment of deep cartilage defects in the knee with autologous chondrocyte transplantation", by Brittberg, Lindahl, Nilsson, Ohlsson, Isaksson, and Peterson, 1994, *The New England Journal of Medicine, 331*, pp. 889-895. Copyright 1994 by the Massachusetts Medical Society. Reprinted with permission.

65% to 70% of 500 joints. Thus, radiation synovectomy appears to be useful as an alternative to surgery for joints that remain refractory to traditional medical management (Deutsch et al., 1993).

Chondrocyte Implantation

Patients with isolated cartilage defects in the femur, tibia, and occasionally the patella are at risk for progressing to OA throughout the knee. Autologous chondrocyte implantation is a new procedure that holds promise for correcting the defect and preventing OA (Brittberg, Lindahl, Nilsson, Ohlsson, Isaksson, & Peterson 1994) (Figure 4). Candidates must be symptomatic and not have arthritis or extensive areas of cartilage damage. In this procedure, cartilage cells are obtained from the healthy femoral condyle during arthroscopy and processed through a special cultivation system. These chondrocytes are placed into the cartilage defect arthroscopically, and a periosteal covering is placed over the cartilage transplant (Brittberg et al., 1994; Minas & Nehrer, 1997). Results are encouraging, but long-term outcomes are unknown.

Postoperative Rehabilitation for Chondrocyte Implantation

The postoperative course is dependent on the site of transplantation, with more caution needed when there is repair of defects on the trochlea and to the patella (Minas & Brigham Orthopedic Associates, 1995). See Table 3 for a postoperative plan.

Table 3. A Postoperative Plan

POD 1

The following procedures are recommended for all transplantation areas:
- CPM machine 0–30°
- Touch-down weight bearing with knee immobilizer
- Immobilizer for sleep
- Ice or Cryocuff™ to the knee
- Quad sets
- Ankle towel roll for full knee extension
- Exercise (femoral defects—passive ROM to active assisted ROM to active ROM of the knee)

POD 2

For femoral condyle or tibial defects
- Advance CPM
- Straight leg raises
- Progress ROM

For patella or trochlear defects
- CPM machine only to 40°
- No straight leg raises
- Passive extension only
- Begin seated or prone active assisted or active ROM
- Flexion only to 90°!

Discharge day

Femoral condyle or tibial defects
- Home CPM machine as tolerated for 3 weeks, 8–12 hr/day
- Touch-down weight bearing
- Immobilizer until independent in staright leg raises
- Immobilizer at night
- Continue active assisted and active ROM and quad sets
- Ice after activity or exercise
- Home physical therapy as needed

Patellar or trochlear defects
- Home CPM 0–40° for 3 weeks, 8–12 hr/day
- Touch-down weight bearing with immobilizer
- Immobilizer at night
- Continue active flexion to 90°
- Passive extension only. No straight leg raises!
- Ice after activity or exercise
- Home physical therapy as needed

ROM goals for both procedures are 90° in 2 weeks and 110° in 4 weeks

At the 4- to 6-week follow-up visit, weight bearing is progressed, and the load is gradually increased as recommended by the surgeon. Muscle strengthening in the static position with weights is usually allowed, as is using the stationary biking with low resistance. Swimming is encouraged with straight-leg kicking only, and this is progressed to aqua jogging.

Between 7 and 12 weeks, crutches may be discontinued if there is sufficient quadriceps control and no gait abnormalities. The type of quadriceps-strengthening exercises used depends on the area of transplantation. Closed-chain activities and balance exercises can be progressed slowly for the femoral and tibial transplants. Isometric training at various angles is safest for patients with patella transplants. Dynamic strengthening should progress slowly.

Cartilage heals slowly, and maturation is complete between 12 and 18 months. A combination of motion, strength, and functional training stimulates healing and integration of the implanted

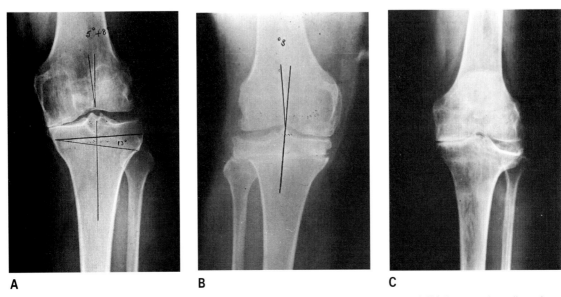

Figure 5. Tibial osteotomy for knee OA (A): Preoperative radiograph with wedge resection illustrated. (B): Postoperative radiograph demonstrating lateral tibial wedge removed with restored valgus alignment. (C): Nine-year postoperative radiograph with mild OA progression and continued excellent function.

tissue, and this is necessary to achieve the best results. Swelling and pain should be avoided, and the program should be reduced if these occur. Light jogging on grass, cross-country skiing, and skating may be possible between 4 and 6 months postoperatively.

Osteotomy

An osteotomy is the surgical removal of bone to realign the joint. In patients in whom OA is present with focal joint destruction of a single joint compartment, an osteotomy can be performed to realign the joint surfaces and shift the load away from the side of the joint that is more arthritic. Because the medial side of the joint is more commonly affected and the knee shifts into a varus alignment, a wedge of bone is removed from the lateral side of the tibia just above the insertion of the patella tendon. The thickness of this lateral tibial wedge will depend on the amount of correction needed to shift the weight from the medial to lateral side of the joint. The goal of the procedure is to put the limb back into its physiological axis of 6° to 8° of valgus alignment. As a general rule, 1 mm of bone is removed from the lateral tibia for every 1° of correction needed. For example, a 10-mm lateral tibial wedge is removed to correct the knee alignment 10°. Therefore, if there is a 5° varus deformity, a wedge of 11 to 12 mm will be removed laterally to shift the knee back into a 6° to 7° valgus alignment (Figure 5).

In patients with lateral compartment arthritis and valgus deformity, wedge osteotomy may still be performed, but the wedge is taken from the supracondylar area of the femur, about 2 in. above the joint line. To bring the knee back into a more varus position and reduce the amount of knee valgus, a medial-based femoral wedge segment of bone is removed. The axis of weight bearing is thereby shifted to the medial and more preserved side of the joint. The amount of bone resected is determined by the degree of deformity, and careful preoperative measurements are made for both tibial and femoral osteotomy to ensure a proper correction of deformity and realignment of the joint surface.

There are strict criteria for selection of patients for osteotomy (Ivarsson & Gillquist, 1991; Ivarsson, Mynerts, & Gillquist, 1990). An osteotomy should be performed only when the damage is localized to one compartment (medial or lateral) and patella femoral pathology is minimal. For this reason, osteotomy is rarely performed in patients with RA. In addition, if there is a major flexion contracture of the knee joint, osteotomy is less successful. The procedure is most suited to younger, active patients or laborers who, because of age or employment, are not ideal candidates for prosthetic replacement.

Recovery from osteotomy is prolonged (3–4 months on average) because the bone from which the wedge has been removed must heal in the same fashion as a fracture would heal. Internal fixation devices are now used routinely to provided immediate stabilization of the osteotomy fragments and thereby allow early joint motion. The use of staples and small plates allows early knee motion without plaster immobilization. Before internal fixation was available, a plaster cast was used after tibial osteotomy, and knee motion was prevented for 6 to 8 weeks.

Postoperative Rehabilitation of Osteotomy

After an osteotomy, weight bearing is protected with crutches for 4 to 8 weeks (longer after femoral osteotomy). As the radiographs demonstrate healing at the osteotomy site, weight bearing is progressed.

Strengthening exercises are begun immediately after surgery, first with isometrics and gradually progressing to a more comprehensive and vigorous resistance program. Physical therapy is required after discharge from the hospital to help the patient increase knee ROM, to improve strength and transfer ability, and to progress ambulation first with external support and then to full weight bearing as healing at the osteotomy site occurs (Ivarsson & Gillquist, 1991).

Swelling and pain may limit the patient's ability to perform antigravity exercises for 2 to 4 weeks after osteotomy. ROM is encouraged early after surgery because stability of the osteotomy fragments has been achieved with internal fixation. A continuous passive motion (CPM) machine can be used postoperatively, and, if there is great limitation of knee motion, it can be continued after hospital discharge. Active assisted motion should be done in the most comfortable position and in one that does not put a medial or lateral stress on the joint. For instance, a varus stress may result from a person overassisting in sidelying exercises (pulling instead of guiding) or from using the uninvolved leg as an assist in the sitting or prone position.

The surgeon may approve the use of a bicycle, without resistance, for early ROM as long as the knee is properly aligned. As healing progresses, resistance is increased, and resistance can be added to stationery biking usually 6 to 8 weeks after the operation.

Results with tibial and femoral osteotomy tend to be good in the short term but often deteriorate over time. The current literature reports 60% to 70% satisfactory function in patients 10 years after osteotomy (Bouharras et al., 1994; Ivarsson et al., 1990; Rudan & Simurda, 1990; Specchiulli, LaForgia, & Solarino, 1990; Stern, Bowen, Insall, & Scuderi, 1990; Yasuda, Majima, Tsuchida, & Kaneda, 1992). Deterioration occurs mostly from progression of OA on the opposite side of the joint. The procedure itself is designed to lessen load on the damaged side of the knee joint, but eventual degradation occurs on the more preserved side of the knee. Knee replacement is feasible after failed osteotomy but is more complex than in a primary knee with OA (Mont, Alexander, et al., 1994; Neyret, Deroche, Deschamps, & Dejour, 1992). The internal fixation must be removed. This requires more extensive dissection around the knee joint, which may lead to problems with soft-tissue healing. Skin healing may be a problem because a different incision is required for the knee replacement. Because an osteotomy requires removal of bony wedges around the knee joint, bony cuts for knee replacement are more complicated, and, on occasion, bone grafts and metal wedges must be attached to the knee implant to deal with bone deficiency produced by the osteotomy. Rehabilitation may be slower because of the more extensive surgery, and outcome may be compromised compared with a primary knee arthroplasty (Ivarsson & Gillquist, 1991). For these reasons, TKA is recommended over osteotomy in less active, younger patients and in older patients with OA of the knee. In patients with inflammatory arthritis, TKA is the procedure of choice because of the more global nature of the disease.

Total Knee Arthroplasty

Total Knee Arthroplasty (TKA) is widely recognized to produce quantifiable benefits for persons with arthritis in reducing pain, improving joint motion and mobility, and enhancing ability to perform activities of daily living (ADL). Additional studies have reported improved sleep, decreased fatigue, decreased depression and anxiety, and overall improvement in quality of life (Bohannon & Cooper, 1993; Drewett, Minns, & Sibly, 1992; Mattson & Weidenhielm, 1995; Pitson, Bhaskaran, Bond, Yarnold, & Drewett, 1994; Rissanen, Seppo, Slatis, Sintonen, & Paavolainen, 1995).

Prosthetic knee replacement is most commonly performed for advanced OA or RA of the knee. The procedure resurfaces the knee and restores physiological alignment to the joint. Relief of pain is expected because all components of the destroyed joint are replaced. Most commonly, three separate components are used: femoral, tibial, and patellar (Figure 6). The femoral component is usually made of a cobalt chrome alloy and closely resembles the normal configuration of the distal femur. The tibial surface that articulates with the metal femoral component is always made of a plastic material called *ultra-high-weight polyethylene*. This may be reinforced with a cobalt chrome tray, or the component may be completely made of polyethylene. The patellar component is polyethylene and is dome-shaped to allow articulation with the groove in the femoral component. By using these three components, all damaged surfaces of the knee joint are covered with new synthetic material, and all arthritic areas are resected. These implants are generally fixed to bone with an acrylic cement called *methylmethacrylate*, which rigidly bonds implant to bone. If bone is well preserved, porous noncemented fixation may be used, but cemented TKA is the preferred technique.

Along with resurfacing, the joint must be realigned to a normal physiological degree of valgus, and ligament stability must be restored. This generally can be accomplished by managing the ligament and soft-tissue asymmetry present about the joint. If soft-tissue symmetry is not accomplished, instability will persist, and the patient may complain of "giving way" or "buckling." Some TKAs may preserve the posterior cruciate ligament, and others have a design that substitutes for it. There is a debate about whether the posterior cruciate ligament is functioning in most cases when it is preserved. It cannot be preserved in severe deformities. In extreme cases when stability cannot be achieved, a more constrained implant may be used. This constrained condylar knee design has increased stability because of a deeper trough in the femoral component into which a longer and

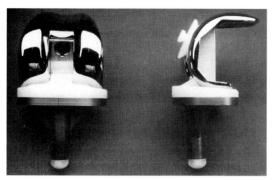

Figure 6. TKA with femoral, tibial, and patella components.

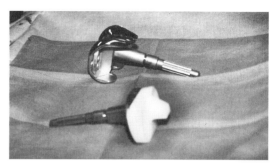

Figure 7. Constrained condylar knee replacement with stems to improve fixation into medullary canals and higher polyethylene peg on tibial component.

thicker peg on the tibial component fits. Medial–lateral and anteroposterior stability is provided by this device and can substitute for deficient ligament support (Figure 7).

For OA. In severe OA with marked deformity, bone loss is common. This generally results from bony impaction with destruction of the femoral condyle or tibial plateau. These areas of bone loss must be augmented either with bone graft taken from bone resected as part of the procedure or with metal augments attached to the prosthesis to fill these areas of bone deficiency (Atchek, Sculco, & Rawlins, 1989). This procedure is necessary in 2% to 3% of patients (Figure 8 and Figure 9). Constrained devices may be necessary because more severely deformed knees often have severe ligamentous incompetence as well as bone deficiency. Bone grafting is likewise performed in the patient with RA who has severe bone loss.

Patients undergoing TKA often donate two units of autologous blood for transfusion during surgery or hospitalization. Knee replacement is usually performed under regional epidural anesthesia and light sedation. Operative time for routine TKA surgery is about 90 min. The epidural catheter may be left in place postoperatively for 1 to 2 days for pain relief.

For inflammatory arthritis. If a patient requires bilateral knee replacements, the procedure can either be scheduled either 5 to 7 days apart or performed sequentially under one anesthesia (Jankiewicz, Sculco, Ranawat, Behr, & Tarrentino, 1994). Performing both replacements at once is particularly useful in patients with severe polyarthritis or severe flexion contracture. Because operative time for knee replacement is in the range of 90 min, both knees can be replaced usually in less than 3 hr. More careful monitoring is required in the perioperative period in these patients.

In patients with RA and hip and knee involvement, the most painful joint is replaced first. If all joints are involved and need replacement, then the hip procedures are performed first and the knees second. In rehabilitation of the knee, care must be taken to prevent dislocation of a recently replaced hip. Preoperative evaluation and discharge planning is extremely important for patients undergoing multiple procedures. Having two or more arthroplasty procedures in one hospitalization is taxing on the patient and the rehabilitation team. Patients must be carefully selected and fully educated preoperatively about what to expect.

Preoperative evaluation. A preoperative evaluation is critical to the outcome of TKA because potential problem areas can be identified at this time (Ganz, 1993). This evaluation allows the physical

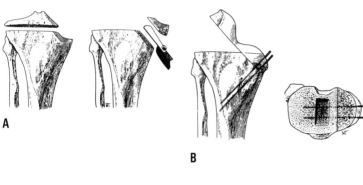

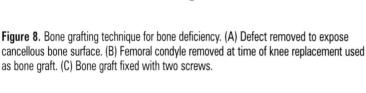

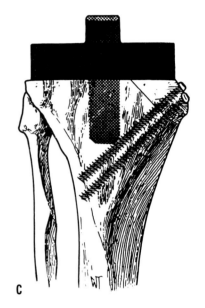

Figure 8. Bone grafting technique for bone deficiency. (A) Defect removed to expose cancellous bone surface. (B) Femoral condyle removed at time of knee replacement used as bone graft. (C) Bone graft fixed with two screws.

therapist to evaluate the patient's gait, posture, and functioning. It allows an opportunity for effective education when the patient's cognitive ability is not clouded by anesthesia, analgesics, pain, or the stress of surgery and hospitalization. Some facilities find preoperative training in ambulation aids to be particularly cost effective, and the effect of this training on reducing length of stay is being investigated. Addressing potential problems at this time can smooth the hospital course and enable the team to plan for appropriate discharge assistance. Although the long-term outcomes are positive, the patient must contend with the immediate postoperative physical problems such as pain, limitations in mobility, and diminished ability to perform ADL independently. The preoperative evaluation is the ideal time to educate the patient on postoperative interventions and help the patient develop realistic expectations of the arthroplasty experience and his or her discharge planning needs. To that end, physical therapy and occupational therapy interventions are vital to assist the patient in achieving his or her highest level of functional independence. Patient education, whether individually or in groups, has been shown to allay fears and enhance short- and long-term outcomes (Lichtenstein, Semaan, & Marmar, 1993; Roach, Trembray, & Bowers, 1995).

In facilities that support preoperative evaluation for TKA, such evaluations are usually done by the physical therapist. Preoperative occupational therapy evaluations are usually only done on patients with severe polyarticular disease. A comprehensive preoperative physical therapy evaluation includes the following:

- *ROM.* ROM of the knee is recorded, and functional ROM of the trunk and other joints is noted.

- *Muscle strength.* Strength testing is performed to determine the weight-bearing abilities of the upper and lower extremities and to determine the type of ambulatory aids necessary during the postoperative period. Manual muscle testing of the quadriceps muscles is typical but is not an indication of function. More objective measures of torque and power can be done with isokinetic systems, but this is neither practical, necessary, nor cost effective in clinical settings.

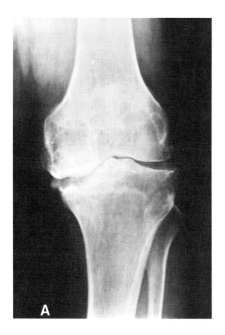
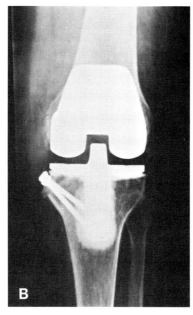

Figure 9. Radiographs of bone grafting technique. (A) Preoperative OA knee with tibial bone deficiency. (B) Five years after bone grafting procedure and TKA.

- *Respiration.* A basic respiratory evaluation includes a cardiorespiratory history, auscultation, and spirometry with a incentive spirometer or blow bottles to determine gross inspiratory and expiratory capacity. These devices are often standard treatment in the early postoperative phase for patients who use general anesthesia or have a history of respiratory problems (Craven, Evans, Davenport, & Williams, 1974; Ganz & Viellion, 1996).

- *Gait.* An observational gait evaluation is performed to determine patient's weight-bearing ability, gait deviations, and patterns on equipment and on level surfaces and stairs. Deviations in cadence, velocity, and single-limb support time can be obtained with a foot-switch stride analyzer (Otis, Fabien, & Burstein, 1983). Pre- and postoperatively, gait studies have been reported in TKA and have shown that both level walking and stair climbing is influenced by the design of the prosthesis (Kettelkamp, Johnson, Smidt, Chao, & Walker, 1970). On ascending stairs, a prosthesis that retains both cruciate ligaments functions closest to normal (Anderson, Andriacchi, & Galante, 1981). Andriacchi, Galante, and Fermier (1982) found that patients with the less-constrained TKA prothestic designs that retained the cruciate ligament had a more normal gait during stair climbing than patients with more constrained cruciate-sacrificing designs. Performance-based measures of gait and balance dysfunction can be obtained easily with the Tinetti Assessment Tool (Appendix 1), which has been shown to be valid and reliable in geriatric patients. The assessment takes approximately 6 to 8 min to perform (Tinetti, 1986; Tinetti & Speechley, 1989).

- *Functional ability.* Functional evaluations are used to monitor progress during hospitalization and to track long-term outcome. The Western Ontario McMaster Universities Osteoarthritis Index (WOMAC; Bellamy, Buchanan, Goldsmith, Campbell, & Stitt, 1988) and the Hospital for Special Surgery Rating Scale (Insall, 1993) are instruments widely used in lower-extremity joint surgery. The WOMAC is a disease-specific tool that measures degree of pain, stiffness, and difficulty with lower-extremity tasks and can be used either in a visual analog format or with word descriptor (see Appendix 2). The questionnaire can be expanded to inquire about each hip and knee. The Medical Outcomes Study Short Form (SF-36) (Ware & Sherbourne, 1992 [see the Appendix at the end of the book]) is a generic assessment of health that is widely used in health care research.

- *Pain.* If pain is to be evaluated, it must be done in a standard fashion. The easiest method is the visual analog scale, which is considered the most reliable and valid way to document subjective pain (Dixon & Bird, 1981; Scott & Huskisson, 1976). Pain intensity may be recorded for specific activities, or a global rating may be obtained. It is important to evaluate the patient's skills and previous training in pain management, such as use of modalities, relaxation techniques, and so forth.

- *Cognition.* Cognitive screening will identify issues that may impair learning and or full participation in the rehabilitation program. This includes orientation, memory, and judgment.

- *Home situation and social support.* Information from a social and environment evaluation is essential to discharge planning. For instance, does the patient live alone? What is the physical environment? Are there stairs? Railings? Are the rooms accessible with ambulatory aids? On what floor are the bedroom and toilet located? Who does the cooking and cleaning, laundry, and grocery shopping? Is there assistance for transportation? If the patient works, what are the demands of the job? What are the leisure pursuits, and what are the physical demands of these activities?

Functional activities critical for discharge planning are:

- the ability to perform lower-extremity dressing, bathing, and foot care;

- the ability to perform safe transfers to and from the bed, chair, toilet, bathtub or shower, and the car;

- use of assistive devices; and

- limitations in activity tolerance or endurance with ADL.

On the basis of the results of the evaluation process, rehabilitation staff members can begin to integrate the information into the treatment planning and discharge process. It should be recognized that the functional, environmental, and social components of this evaluation can be a helpful predictor of discharge disposition. In a study of 162 patients with total hip and knee replacements, patients who lived alone were more likely to be discharged to a rehabilitation unit than to home. In addition, these patients requiring rehabilitation placement were older and had more than two comorbid conditions (Munin, Kwoh, Glynn, Crossett, & Rubash, 1995).

Postoperative Rehabilitation for TKA. Because the first TKA was performed more than 30 years ago, methods and philosophies of rehabilitation have changed, yet the primary goal has remained the same—to provide a pain free, stable joint with a functional ROM. This means $0°$ extension and $90°$ flexion that the patient can maintain easily that is sufficient for ADL.

Twenty years ago, patients were hospitalized for 2 to 3 weeks for each knee and may have been casted for 7 to 10 days before flexion was initiated. Today, flexion is initiated within 24 hr postoperatively, and often a CPM machine is used (Figure 10). Average length of stay for an uncomplicated TKA is 5 to 7 days, and some institutions plan on decreasing it to 4 days if discharge plans are adequate (Coutts, Kaita, & Barr, 1982; Ganz, 1993). Table 3 shows a sample clinical pathway, and Appendix 3 shows a multidisciplinary documentation form for TKE. Appendix 4 is a sample patient and

family member version of a clinical pathway.

Immediate postoperative care. The
patient may return from the
recovery room either with a
CPM machine, a knee immobilizer, or a primary bulky dressing.
Cryotherapy is usual, with some
facilities using ice and others
using the Cryocuff™ units for
cooling and compression. Pneumatic boots for venous compression are many surgeons' preference and are typically used until
the patient is ambulatory.

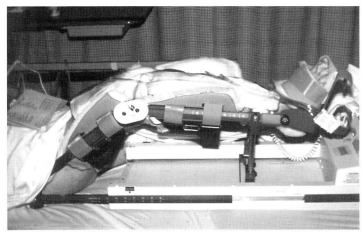

Figure 10. Patient positioned in a CPM machine.

Most patients will have some type of drainage apparatus (hemovac) in the knee. Approximately 200 ml of serous drainage is expected to collect during the first 8 hr (Smeltzer & Bare,
1992). Accumulation will decrease to less than 25 ml per 24-hr period before the apparatus is
removed.

Bed mobility is limited for most patients because of the CPM machine, intravenous catheter,
and urinary catheter. Those who have an epidural catheter in place for pain control will be unable to
move the legs, so attention to skin integrity is essential. Positioning and pressure areas should be
checked every 2 hr. Postoperative pain may be managed with a patient-controlled analgesia pump or
by intramuscular injection. Peroneal nerve injury occurs in 3% to 4% of patients after TKA and
most often in persons who have had epidural anesthesia and epidural postoperative pain management (Idusuyi & Morrey, 1996). By the second postoperative day, oral analgesics are used and timed
to be given 30 min before therapy.

CPM. The CPM machine passively flexes and extends the knee at a designated speed and arc of
motion that is set or programmed by the physical therapist, nurse, or physician. Studies on the benefits and drawbacks of the CPM machine have been mixed. Some studies indicate that CPM may be
beneficial in counteracting the effect of joint immobilization by improving postoperative venous
flow and in maintenance of articular cartilage nutrition (Coutts et al., 1982; Goetz & Rand, 1988;
Salter, Clements, & Ogilivie-Harris, 1982). A multinstitutional study (Coutts et al., 1982) of postoperative TKA treatment found a more rapid gain in knee motion after TKA coupled with decreased
length of stay for patients who received CPM therapy compared with a control group. Other studies concur (Gose, 1987; Jordan, Siegel, & Olivo, 1995). However, in similar controlled designs, no
great differences in ROM at discharge were found with CPM therapy compared with conventional
physical therapy (Kumar, McPherson, Door, Wan, & Baldwin, 1996; Montgomery & Eliasson, 1996;
Ritter, Gandolf, & Holston, 1989). Ritter and colleagues (1989) further concluded that knees treated with CPM were weaker, had greater extensor lags, and appeared to have less ambulatory
endurance as a result of confinement in bed to allow use of the CPM machine. A decreased incidence of deep-vein thrombosis has been reported by Kim and Moon (1995), yet Rand (1991)

Table 3. Sample Clinical Pathway

Hospital for Special Surgery TKA Clinical Pathway

DAY OF SURGERY 5N → OR → PACU → INPT.	POD1	POD2	POD 3	POD 4	POD 5	POD 6
Verify H&P ortho exam Ortho exam Review data base Anesthesia Pain service Pastoral care Dietician	Social work screen	→	Reassess need for home care/ rehabilitation/ extended care/ placement/ counseling	Confirm discharge plan	Finalize discharge plan/transportation with patient/family/team	D/C
Type and cross	Lytes, H&H PT daily if on Coumadin	Lytes, H&H	Lytes, H&H			
Antibiotic 1 hr prior to incision/continue x 24 hr Pain, IM or PCA	Antibiotic D/C Pain, IM or PCA DVT Prophylaxis • Coumadin • ASA Routine meds, PRNs	Wean to PO		Anticipate coumadin for home	Instructions for home meds	
N.P.O. → Clear based on bowel sounds	Clear liquids	Progress to regular as tolerated		Regular diet		
M.D. admitting orders • Skin prep • Prep • Shave • IV • Foley • Compression device • O₂ • Drains				TED'S Incentive Inspirometer Ambulate 2 to 3x Logroll OOB for meals		

Table 3. (cont.)

Hospital for Special Surgery TKA Clinical Pathway

DAY OF SURGERY 5N → OR → PACU → INPT.	POD1	POD2	POD 3	POD 4	POD 5	POD 6
Comfort measures *Initiate Standard Orders:* • Postop • Pain • Nursing care plan. TKR	Continue and individualize standard orders					
Initiate Nursing Protocols: • Management of Pt in SDS OR PACU • Acute Pain, PCA, Jr IM • Postop major ortho • Elimination	Continue and individualize protocols	D/C, PCA D/C IV/I&O D/C/ Foley	Pain <3/10	Pain <3/10	Pain <3/10	Pain <3/10
Initiate Physical Therapy Initiate CPM in PACU 0-60 ↑ as tolerated	*Physical Therapy* —AROM —↑ CPM as tolerated —Transfer training —Ambulation with walker (WBAT)		*PT* ↑ROM as tolerated advance to cane as tolerated	Pain <3/10 instructions on stairs Home exercise program	review stairs review home program	

Note. From the Hospital for Special Surgery, New York, NY. Reprinted with permission.

reached contradicting results regarding the effects on swelling and blood loss. Contraindications to CPM use include:

- sensory deficits excluding epidural anesthesia,
- excessive wound drainage,
- postoperative confusion and delirium, and
- prothrombin time of greater than 22 sec and an international normalized ration of greater than 3 (Ortel, 1995).

Patients whose active extension is poor and who concomitantly have a flexion contracture should have limited time in the CPM machine with aggressive therapy to improve knee extension. For this purpose, a dynamic knee brace may be indicated (Ganz, 1993). Follow-up studies at intervals varying from a few weeks to 2 years found no major ROM differences related to CPM machine use (Ritter et al., 1989; Ververeli, Sutton, Hearn, & Booth, 1995), whereas Johnson and Eastwood (1992) found greater knee motion at 1 year postoperatively. Contrary to these findings, Kim and Moon (1995) studied ROM in the squatting position with ROM measured at 3.5 years postoperatively and found that the group that did not use CPM had much greater flexion. McInnes and colleagues (1992) concluded that CPM use decreased the need for manipulation after TKA, which is a costly and painful procedure. They likewise found no difference in ROM at 6 months and at 2 years between the groups using and not using the CPM machine (McInnes et al., 1992; Ververeli et al., 1995). Despite the limitations reported for CPM therapy, surgeons at The Hospital for Special Surgery (New York, NY) and Brigham and Women's Hospital (Boston, MA) believe the benefits outweigh the drawbacks, and they currently use the CPM machines.

CPM application and use is determined by the philosophy of the institution and the surgeon because outcome data are still conflicting. If the CPM is applied in the recovery room, the primary compression dressing dictates the degree at which the CPM machine should be set. When the dressing is bulky, the CPM machine is set at a lower ROM (0° to 45°). Bulky dressings kink and create pressure areas on the posterior surface of the knee at higher degrees of motion. If the compression dressing is thin, the degrees may be set to 90° (Ganz, 1993; Jordan et al., 1995). Some physicians do not recommend use of the CPM machine until the first postoperative day because its use with the freshly cut bone combines to produce excessive bleeding during the first 24 hr postoperatively.

CPM is increased to the patient's tolerance. It is critical that all staff members have a thorough understanding of the mechanics of CPM and the proper placement of the limb in the machine. Through preoperative teaching, the patient is made aware of the proper use of the CPM machine and the need to combine functional activities to gain the knee flexion required for ADL.

Initiation of transfer activities, gait training, and active ROM are usually begun on the first postoperative day and continued until the patient is discharged or achieves 90° flexion. There is no consensus regarding discharge to home with a CPM machine. CPM should be considered when the patient is having difficulty with flexion and the interoperative measurement indicates that motion is possible.

Gait training. There is consensus regarding weight-bearing status after a cemented or uncemented TKA. Some protocols promote partial weight bearing with two crutches, and others allow full weight bearing with a cane. There is concern that early postoperative weight bearing can result in implant loosening, but there are no prospective randomized controlled trials that examine this issue.

Patients are advanced from a walker to crutches to a cane, depending on their functional abilities, the status of other joints, and the surgeon's guidelines. Many surgeons tend toward conservative progression of ambulation because soft tissue takes approximately 6 weeks to heal. Activity such as walking on a weak quadriceps muscle without an assistive device can increase swelling and stress soft-tissue repair, so it is discouraged.

Some facilities discharge the patient with one crutch or cane, but most patients are discharged with two crutches or a walker, particularly if discharge to a rehabilitation facility is planned. By 6 weeks, most patients have progressed to needing only one crutch or a cane for outdoor activities. The patient should not be hasty in discontinuing the device. If gait is antalgic (not smooth), then the device should be used, particularly for long walks. It is better from a cardiorespiratory point of view to use a cane and walk further than to keep the distance short because of muscular weakness or general fatigue.

Exercise for motion and function. Factors that influence postoperative ROM are prosthetic design, preoperative deformity, and intraoperative bone resection (Ganz, 1993). Early postoperative motion will be influenced by the degree of swelling and soft-tissue procedures. The practitioner should be aware of the ROM obtained during surgery and should include ROM as a goal in the discharge plans. Therapy is aimed at increasing active flexion for the requirements of ADL. Kettelkamp and colleagues (1970) have documented the average ROM used for selected functional tasks with electromyographic studies (Table 4).

Most hospital exercise programs typically consist of:

- passive, assisted, and active ROM;
- quadriceps and hamstring isometric strengthening exercises; and
- open- and closed-chain ROM and strengthening.

Table 4. Average Knee ROM Demonstrated During Functional Activities

ADL Mean Knee ROM	
Walking (swing phase)	67°
Ascending stairs	83°
Descending stairs	90°
Rising from chair	93°
Tying shoe	106°
Lifting object off floor	117°

Source: "An Electrogoniometric Study of Knee Motion in Normal Gait," by D. B. Kettelkamp, 1970, *Journal of Bone and Joint Surgery, 52A*, pp. 775–790; and "A Quantitative Analysis of Knee Motion During Activities of Daily Living," by K. N. Laubenthal, G. L. Smidt, and D. B. Kettelkamp, 1972, *Physical Therapy, 52*, pp. 34–42.

Some institution protocols include

- straight-leg raising and possibly short-arc quadriceps exercises (terminal knee extension exercises) from 30° to 0°,
- patella mobilization as needed, and
- stationary biking or restorator.

Because of the shortened length of hospitalization, bikes are more often used at home, in rehabilitation units, and in outpatient clinics. At the Robert B. Brigham Hospital (Boston, MA) in the 1970s and early 1980s, all patients were encouraged to purchase bicycles, and bike progression protocols were developed. Bikes with chains or belts that allow smooth backward rocking and revolutions are easier to use, particularly in the early stage of motion.

Exercises for strengthening. Progression of the strengthening program varies. Some surgeons allow the use of ankle weights and Theraband™ (Hygenic Corp., Akron, OH) beginning at 2 weeks; others do not allow use of these devices for 1 to 3 months. Most surgeons make recommendations on an individual basis, including resistance on the bike and isokinetic

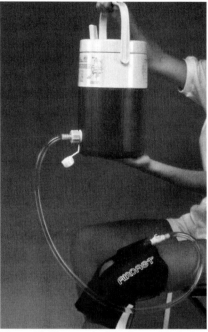

Figure 11. Photograph of the Cryocuff™ device for cooling the knee.

work in a therapeutic or recreational setting. The patient should ask the surgeon specific questions on exercise and recreation because many physicians do not automatically discuss them.

Modalities. Cryotherapy in the form of a Cryocuff™ device, ice, or cold packs are often used immediately postoperatively and always after exercise sessions to decrease and minimize swelling. Heat can increase swelling in the joint, and it should be avoided (Figure 11).

Functional electrical stimulation (FES) to the quadriceps can assist the strengthening process and decrease the extensor lag. An extensor lag (the inability to actively extend the knee to 0° when passively achieved) is often seen after TKA, particularly in patients who have used the CPM machine. Haug and Wood (1988) examined the effectiveness of neuromuscular stimulation of the quadriceps muscles after TKA and concluded that CPM combined with FES is a worthwhile adjunctive therapy when muscle reeducation is needed. Transcutaneous electrical nerve stimulation may be used in conjunction with cold modalities for patients in whom pain is difficult to manage by medication alone and for patients who are having a difficult time achieving flexion (Ganz, 1993).

Inpatient functional milestones. An important aspect of TKA rehabilitation is the ability to measure functional milestones during hospitalization. After surgery, the patient's level of activity rapidly increases. This improvement in function must occur despite chronic shortages in hospital staff members and fiscal constraints. It is necessary to carefully measure functional progression to ensure that patients achieve specific functional milestones in a timely fashion. By consensual agreement of the inpatient staff members at The Hospital for Special Surgery, a functional progression for TKA patients was developed (seeTable 5). This functional milestone form has proven to be a valid and reliable tool (Kroll et al., 1994) to determine the mean postoperative day of achievement of specific

Table 5. Unilateral Uncomplicated TKA POD of Achievement of Functional Milestones (*N*=600)

Functional Milestone	Mean POD of Achievement	Standard Deviation
Walker unassisted	5.2	1.82
Transfer unassisted	5.2	1.73
Stairs unassisted	6.5	1.93
POD @90	6.8	1.87
POD of discharge	6.1	2.64
	8.1	2.43

Note. From the Hospital for Special Surgery, New York, NY. Reprinted with permission.

functional milestones that patients are required to achieve before discharge from the hospital. Specific functional milestones addressed are transfers in and out of bed, walker use, cane use, stair ambulation, active knee ROM, and postoperative day of discharge. The milestones are characterized by two levels of achievement: assisted and unassisted. Assisted achievement is defined as that requiring assistance from another person to perform the task, which includes manual assistance, contact guarding, verbal cuing, and supervision. The use of an ambulatory aid is not considered assisted because every patient is discharged with an ambulatory aid.

ADL and assistive devices. The primary focus of occupational therapy is to provide the patient with tools and skills to regain functional independence in ADL postoperatively. For patients with monoarticular involvement, the initial limitations are the inability to fully flex the knee and limited weight bearing on the operated extremity. These factors contribute to difficulty with lower-extremity self-care, transfers, and ambulation.

Training in the use of assistive devices such as a long-handled sponge for bathing, a sock aid, and a hooked dressing stick should be provided on the basis of individual need and desire to attain independence. In addition, elevated toilet seats or shower stools for the bathtub may be necessary. The Abledata database (www.abledata.com) contains complete current listings and purchasing information for all adaptive equipment.

It is imperative that the clinician be aware of the guidelines for weight bearing. Patient use of aids should be observed by the occupational therapy practitioner, and proper, safe techniques should be reinforced in all aspects of ADL. It is important to note that patients with monoarticular disease often do not require lower-extremity self-care aids because they can substitute hip motion for limited mobility of the knee in the early postoperative phase (Melvin, 1989). Patients with polyarticular involvement may be more likely to require assistive devices until full mobility is achieved. Individual surgeon protocols may influence the use of assistive devices. Some may be concerned that use of or reliance on devices may limit postoperative flexion and therefore do not approve of their use.

Sports and driving. The most common cause of failure in TKA is mechanical loosening. By placing undue force on the knee joint, the patient increases the chance of prosthetic loosening and endangers the overall success of the knee replacement (Insall, 1993). Patients are often instructed before and after surgery to avoid sports that would place excessive force on the prosthetic knee joint (e.g., running, jumping, singles tennis). Golf has been considered to be a safe sport. More than 95% of orthopedic surgeons who are members of The Knee Society allow their patients to play golf. But

Mallon and Callaghan (1993) studied the effects of golf on TKA and found that radiographic lucent lines occurred in 79.1% of cemented arthroplasties, 49% of uncemented arthroplasties, and 53.9% of all TKAs studied. Pain rates during and after play were much higher in golfers with left TKAs than for those with right TKAs. It is believed that this is a direct result of increased torque on the left knee in right-handed golfers. The use a golf cart is definitely recommended.

"When can I resume driving?" is often asked even before surgery. Spalding, Kiss, and Kyberd (1994) studied the driving reaction time of 40 patients with right TKAs and found that the driving reaction time did not return to normal until approximately 8 weeks after surgery. Patients with left TKAs did not have impaired ability to brake. Even if the patient's car has automatic transmission, most surgeons do not allow driving until after the 4- to 6-week checkup because of soft-tissue healing and the effects of pain medications.

Joint protection. A common misconception is that, once a joint is replaced, it is as good as new. It should be stressed to the patient that the prosthetic replacement is not a normal joint and must be protected even when pain abates and ROM and function improve. TKA patients should be counseled to maintain a healthy weight and to reduce unnecessary stress to the implant, which may contribute to accelerated loosening of the components. The patient must be willing to participate in an exercise program to strengthen the surrounding musculature, use aids as needed for temporary protection of the joint, and observe the postoperative precautions. Joint protection principles that diminish extraneous forces on the knee implant include, but are not limited to,

- sitting to perform ADL such as dressing, bathing, and meal preparation;
- avoiding kneeling on hands and knees for gardening or cleaning the floors or the bathtub;
- using a small gardening stool and long-handled mops, sponges, and brushes;
- avoiding unnecessary stairs; and
- avoiding prolonged periods of standing (sit and take a break when possible).

Home Health Care and Outpatient Services

Patients undergoing unilateral knee replacement are usually discharged home between 4 and 7 days postoperatively. Often patients with systemic disease or those who have multiple joint procedures performed at the same time will require transitional placement in a rehabilitation facility or a skilled nursing facility until ADL can be done safely. With the advent of managed care, many patients have either hospital case managers or insurance case managers. This person should coordinate the discharge plans. It is the practitioner's responsibility to customize the home exercise program so that the patient can work toward maximizing function. The number of visits by or to a practitioner is determined not only by documentation of progress but also by insurance guidelines. The patient must work toward gaining a functional degree of flexion necessary to perform basic ADL before progressing to the strengthening program. Common questions for practitioner are:

- *How do I progress the bike at home?* With 75° to 80° of flexion, good control from the other foot, and adequate seat height, rocking on the bike to increase motion is possible, but revolutions are not. The emphasis should be hip flexion rather than knee flexion because often the patient contracts the quadriceps muscles when the motion is painful. Generally, 90° to 100° of comfortable motion is necessary to ride forward and backward without compensation from other joints (i.e., leaning to opposite side and hiking the hip). There usually are no precautions with biking as in hip arthroplasty other than to minimize pain and swelling. Lowering the bike seat as motion increases is encouraged but only to the point considered to be normal biking position of the knee. Increasing to 10 to 30 min a day is encouraged. This will depend on the status of the other joints and on whether the person is using the bike for cardiovascular activity. Light to moderate tension is usually allowed, but the patient should clear this with the surgeon.

- *When should the knee immobilizer be used?* Most often, the immobilizer is used at night during the early postoperative phase (1–3 weeks) to increase and maintain knee extension. It is used during ambulation when the patient has insufficient quadriceps control to maintain the knee in extension. If a contracture existed, then the immobilizer may need to be straightened out as the extension improves. Instructing the patient in prone lying (i.e., feet or entire leg off the end of the bed) is an excellent method of passive stretching. In the sitting or supine position, a folded ankle roll can be used throughout the day to stretch the posterior soft tissues.

- *When is exercising in water allowed?* Most surgeons do not allow aquatic exercise for at least 5 to 7 days postoperatively. (Showering is allowed.) If aquatic therapy is an option in the first few weeks, then the patient is usually under the supervision of a practitioner. The patient should be cautioned against returning to his or her recreational pool before the first postoperative visit and until crutches are discontinued. Surgeon approval is recommended if the aquatic exercise is not under the guidance of a practitioner.

Outcome and Complications

The reported long-term results of TKA have been excellent. Most series document at least 90% good to excellent results at minimum 10-year follow-up. (Buechel & Pappas, 1989; Insall, 1993; Ranawat, Flynn, Saddler, Hansraj, & Maynard, 1993; Stern et al., 1990; Stern & Insall, 1992). Mechanical loosening has been uncommon. Most failures have been related to design problems with thin polyethylene surfaces or implants that produce excessive loading to the polyethylene surfaces. Should failure occur, revision knee replacement surgery is usually performed.

Infection remains the most catastrophic complication after knee replacement. Deep periprosthetic infection occurs in less than 1% of patients. Bacterial infiltration occurs rapidly in the bone cement or bone implant interface, and this makes eradication of the infection impossible without removal of the implant and all foreign material. A 6-week course of parenteral antibiotics is administered intravenously, and then reimplantation of the knee is performed (Windsor, Insall, Urs, Miller, & Brause, 1990). Various designs of spacers to fill the void after implant removal have been tried in an attempt to maintain motion after implant removal. Regardless of when reimplantation is performed, at 6 weeks after implant removal, severe soft-tissue contractures may be present that make ROM difficult. Loss of motion is therefore common after treatment of an infected knee replacement.

Overall, results after reimplantation for knee replacement infection have been encouraging. In a large series of patients from The Hospital for Special Surgery, recurrence rate of infection was less than 5%. Function was compromised by loss of motion, and recovery was prolonged. Patients are more prone to develop myositis ossificans after infection and surgical treatment for it, and this further reduces ultimate knee motion.

Summary

The knee joint is a complex series of interlocking articular surfaces with passive and active soft-tissue constraints and mobilizers. In defining the pathological state of the knee joint when it is symptomatic, all elements of this mechanism must be considered. Furthermore, it is rare that just one component of the knee joint is problematic without some interplay of the adjacent structures. The musculoskeletal physician, surgeon, and physical therapist must recognize the complex interaction and the importance of the soft tissues in functional performance. Rehabilitation plays a pivotal role both in the conservative and surgical management of the knee joint. The orthopedic surgeon and the rehabilitation team must work closely together if postoperative goals are to be achieved.

References

Altchek, D., Sculco, T. P., & Rawlins, B. (1989). Autogenous bone grafting for severe angular deformity in total knee arthroplasty. *Journal of Arthroplasty, 4*, 151–155.

Anderson, G., Andriacchi, T. P., & Galante, J. O. (1981). Correlations between changes in gait and in clinical status after knee arthroplasty. *Acta Orthopaedica Scandinavica, 52*, 569.

Andriacchi, T. P., Galante, J. O., & Fermier, R. W. (1982). The influence of total knee replacement design in walking and stair-climbing. *Journal of Bone and Joint Surgery, 64A*, 1235.

Bellamy, N., Buchanan, W. W., Goldsmith, C. H., Campbell, J., & Stitt, L. (1988). Validation study of the WOMAC: A health status instrument for measuring clinically important patient relevant outcomes to anti-rheumatic drug therapy in patients with osteoarthritis of the hip or knee. *Journal of Rheumatology, 15*, 1833–1840.

Bohannon, R. W., & Cooper, J. (1993). Total knee arthroplasty: Evaluation of an acute care rehabilitation program. *Archives of Physical Medicine and Rehabilitation, 74*, 1091–1094.

Bouharras, M., Hoet, F., Watillon, M., Despontin, J., Geulette, R., Thomas, P., & Parmentier, D. (1994). Results of tibial valgus osteotomy for internal femoro-tibial arthritis with an average 8-year follow-up. *Acta Orthopaedica Belgica, 60*(2), 163–169.

Brittberg, M., Lindahl, A., Nilsson, A., Ohlsson, C., Isaksson, O., & Peterson, L. (1994). Treatment of deep cartilage defects in the knee with autologous chondrocyte transplantation. *Journal of the American Medical Association, 33*, 858–894.

Buechel, F. F., & Pappas, M. J. (1989). New Jersey low contact stress knee replacement system: Ten-year evaluation of meniscal bearings. *Orthopedic Clinics of North America, 20*(2), 147–177.

Convery, F. R., Lyon, R., & Laverna, C. (1994). Uncommon arthropathies: Synovial tumors. In J. H. Klippel & P. A. Dieppe (Eds.), *Rheumatology* (pp. 3.39.1–3.39.8). St. Louis, MO: Mosby.

Coutts, R. D., Kaita, J., & Barr, R. (1982). The role of continuous passive motion in the preoperative rehabilitation of the knee. *Orthopedic Transcripts, 6*, 277.

Craven, J. L., Evans, G. A., Davenport, P. J., & Williams, R. H. (1974). The evaluation of the incentive spirometer in the management of post operative pulmonary complications. *British Journal of Surgery, 61*(10), 793–797.

Deutsch, E., Brodack, J., & Deutsch, K. (1993). Radiation synovectomy revisited. *European Journal of Nuclear Medicine, 20*, 1113–1127.

Dixon, J. S., & Bird, H. A. (1981). Reproducibility along a 10 cm vertical visual analogue scale. *Annals of Rheumatic Diseases, 40*, 87–89.

Drewett, R. F., Minns, R. J., & Sibly, T. F. (1992). Measuring outcome of total knee replacement using quality of life indices. *Annals of the Royal College of Surgeons of England, 74*, 286–290.

Dunscombe, P. R., Bhattacharyya, A. K., & Dale, R. G. (1976). The assessment of the body distribution of yttrium-90 ferric hydroxide during radiation synovectomy. *British Journal of Radiology, 49*, 372–373.

Dunscombe, P. R., & Ramsey, N. W. (1980). Radioactivity studies on 2 synovial specimens after radiation synovectomy with yttrium-90 silicate. *Annals of Rheumatic Diseases, 39*, 87–89.

Ganz, S. B. (1993). Physical therapy of the knee. In J. N. Insall, R. E. Windsor, W. N. Scott, M. A. Kelly, & P. Aglietti (Eds.), *Surgery of the knee* (pp. 1171–1192). New York: Churchill Livingstone.

Ganz, S. B., & Viellion, G. (1996). Pre and post surgical management of the hip and knee. In S. T. Wegener & B. B. Belza (Eds.), *Clinical care in the rheumatic diseases* (pp. 103–106). Atlanta, GA: American College of Rheumatology.

Gibson, J. N., White, M. D., Chapman, V. M., & Strachan, R. K. (1992). Arthroscopic lavage and debridement for osteoarthritis of the knee. *Journal of Bone and Joint Surgery, 74B*, 534–537.

Goetz, D. W., & Rand, J. A. (1988). The role of continuous passive motion following total knee arthroplasty. *Clinical Orthopaedics and Related Research, 226*, 34–37.

Gose, J. C. (1987). CPM in the postoperative treatment of patients with total knee replacement: A retrospective study. *Physical Therapy, 67*, 39.

Haug, J., & Wood, L. T. (1988). Efficacy of neuromuscular stimulation of the quadriceps femoris during continuous passive motion following total knee replacement arthroplasty. *Archives of Physical Medicine Rehabilitation, 69*, 423.

Hochberg, M. C., Altman, R. D., Brandt, K. D., Clark, B. M., Dieppe, P. A., Griffin, M. R., Moskowitz, R. W., & Schnitzer, T. J. (1995). Guidelines for the medical management of osteoarthritis. *Arthritis and Rheumatism, 38*(11), 1541–1546.

Huo, M. H., & Galloway, M. T. (1994). Orthopedic management of the knee in rheumatic diseases. In J. H. Klippel & P. A. Dieppe (Eds.), *Rheumatology* (pp. 8:25.1–8:25.8). St. Louis, MO: Mosby.

Idusuyi, O. B., & Morrey, B. F. (1996). Peroneal nerve palsy after total knee arthroplasty: Assessment of predisposing and prognosis factors. *Journal of Bone and Joint Surgery, 78A*, 177–184.

Insall, J. N. (1993). Bone grafting in total knee replacement. In J. N. Insall, R. E. Windsor, W. N. Scott, M. A. Kelly, & P. Aglietti (Eds.), *Surgery of the knee* (2nd ed.). New York: Churchill Livingstone.

Insall, J. N., Hood, R. W., Flawn, L. B., & Sullivan, D. J. (1983). The total condylar knee prothesis in gonarthrosis: A five to nine year follow-up of the first one hundred consecutive replacements. *Journal of Bone and Joint Surgery, 65A*, 619–628.

Ivarsson, I., & Gillquist, J. (1991). Rehabilitation after high tibial osteotomy and unicompartmental arthroplasty: A comparative study. *Clinical Orthopaedics and Related Research, 266*, 139–144.

Ivarsson, I., Myrnerts, R., & Gillquist, J. (1990). High tibial osteotomy for medial osteoarthritis of the knee: A 5 to 7 and 11 year follow-up. *Journal of Bone and Joint Surgery, 72A*, 238–244.

Jankiewicz, J. J., Sculco, T. P., Ranawat, C. S., Behr, C., & Tarrentino, S. (1994). One-stage versus 2-stage bilateral total knee arthroplasty. *Clinical Orthopaedics and Related Research, 309*, 94–101.

Johnson, D. P., & Eastwood, D. M. (1992). Beneficial effects of continuous passive motion after total condylar knee arthroplasty. *Annals of the Royal College of Surgery, 74*(6), 412–416.

Jette, A. M. (1980). The functional status index: Reliability of a chronic disease evaluation instrument. *Archives of Physical Medicine & Rehabilitation, 61*, 395–401.

Jordan, L. R., Siegel, J. L., & Olivo, J. L. (1995). Early flexion routine: An alternative method of continuous passive motion. *Clinical Orthopaedics and Related Research, 315*, 231–233.

Kettelkamp, D. B., Johnson, R. J., Smidt, G. L., Chao, E. Y., & Walker, M. (1970). An electrogoniometric study of knee motion in normal gait. *Journal of Bone and Joint Surgery, 52A,* 775–790.

Kim, J. M., & Moon, M. S. (1995). Squatting following total knee arthroplasty. *Clinical Orthopaedics and Related Research, 313,* 177–186.

Kroll, M. A., Ganz, S. B., Backus, S. I., Benick, R. A., Mackenzie, C., & Harris, L. (1994). A scale for measuring functional outcomes after total joint arthroplasty. *Arthritis Care and Research, 7,* 78–84.

Kumar, P. J., McPherson, E. J., Door, L. D., Wan, Z., & Baldwin, K. (1996). Rehabilitation after total knee arthroplasty: A comparison of 2 rehabilitation techniques. *Clinical Orthopedics and Related Research, 331,* 93–101.

Laurin, C. A., Desmarchais, J., Daziano, L., Gariepy, R., & Derome, A. (1974). Long-term results of synovectomy of the knee in rheumatoid arthritis. *Journal of Bone and Joint Surgery, 56A,* 521–531.

Lichtenstein, R., Semaan, S., & Marmar, E. C. (1993). Development and impact of a hospital-based perioperative patient education program in a joint replacement center. *Orthopaedic Nursing, 12*(6), 17–25.

Mallon, W. J., & Callaghan, J. J. (1993). Total knee arthroplasty in active golfers. *Journal of Arthroplasty, 8,* 299–306.

Mattsson, E., & Weidenhielm, L. (1995). Improvement after surgery in patients with osteoarthrosis of the knee. *Scandinavian Journal of Caring Science, 9,* 47–54.

McInnes, J., Larson, M. G., Daltroy, L. D., Brown, T., Fossel, A. H., Eaton, H. M., Shulman-Kirwan, B., Steindorf, S., Ross, R., & Liang, M. H. (1992). A controlled evaluation of continuous passive motion in patients undergoing total knee arthroplasty. *Journal of the American Medical Association, 268,* 1423–1428.

McLaren, A. C., Blokker, C. P., Fowler, P. J., Roth, J. N., & Rock, M. G. (1991). Arthroscopic debridement of the knee for osteoarthrosis. *Canadian Journal of Surgery, 34*(6), 595–598.

Meehan, R. F. (1992). The AIMS approach to health status measurement: Conceptual background and measurement properties. *Journal of Rheumatology, 9,* 785–788.

Melvin, J. (Ed.). (1989). *Rheumatic disease in adult and child: Occupational therapy and rehabilitation.* Philadelphia: F. A. Davis.

Minas, T., & Brigham Orthopedic Associates. (1995). *Postoperative protocol for chondrocyte implantation.* Patient education material developed from rehabilitation protocols from the Gottenberg Sweden Medical Center, Gottenberg, Sweden.

Minas, T., & Nehrer, S. (1997). Current concepts in the treatment of articular cartilage defects. *Orthopedics, 26,* 525–538.

Minor, M. (1998). Exercise for health and physical fitness. In J. L. Melvin & G. Jensen (Eds.), *Rheumatologic rehabilitation series. Volume 1. Assessment and management.* Bethesda, MD: American Occupational Therapy Association.

Mont, M. A., Alexander, N., Krackow, K. A., & Hungerford, D. S. (1994). Total knee arthroplasty after failed high tibial osteotomy. *Orthopedic Clinics of North America, 25*(3), 515–525.

Mont, M. A., Antonaides, S., Krackow, K. A., & Hungerford, D. S. (1994). Total knee arthroplasty after failed high tibial osteotomy: A comparison with a matched group. *Clinical Orthopaedics and Related Research, 299,* 125–130.

Montgomery, F., & Eliasson, M. (1996). Continuous passive motion compared to active physical therapy after total knee arthroplasty: Similar hospitalization times in a randomized study of 68 patients. *Acta Orthopaedica Scandinavica, 67,* 709.

Munin, M. C., Kwoh, C. K., Glynn, N., Crossett, L., & Rubash, H. E. (1995). Predicting a discharge outcome after elective hip and knee arthroplasty. *American Journal of Physical Medicine and Rehabilitation, 74*, 294–301.

Neyret, P., Deroche, P., Deschamps, G., & Dejour, H. (1992). [Total knee replacement after valgus tibial osteotomy: Technical problems]. *Revue de Chirurgie Orthopedique et Reparatrice de l'Appareil Moteur, 78*(7), 438–448.

Novak, P. J., & Bach, B. R. Jr. (1993). Selection criteria for knee arthroscopy in the osteoarthritic patient. *Orthopedic Review, 22*(7), 798–804.

Ogilvie-Harris, D. J., & Fitsialos, D. P. (1991). Arthroscopic management of the degenerative knee. *Arthroscopy, 7*(2), 151–157.

Ogilvie-Harris, D. J., & Weisleder, L. (1995). Arthroscopic synovectomy of the knee: Is it helpful? *Arthroscopy, 11*(1), 91–95.

Ortel, L. B. (1995). International normalized ratio (NR): An approved way to monitor oral anticoagulant therapy. *Nurse Practitioner, 20*, 15–22.

Otis, J. C., Fabian, D. F., & Burstein, A. H. (1983). Evaluation of total knee arthroplasty patients using the VA Rancho Gait Analyzer. In H. Matsui & K. Kobayashi (Eds.), *Biomechanics VIII-B* (pp. 1075–1080). Champaign, IL: Human Kinetics.

Pitson, D., Bhaskaran, V., Bond, H., Yarnold, R., & Drewett, R. (1994). Effectiveness of knee replacement surgery in arthritis. *International Journal of Nursing Studies, 3*, 49–56.

Ranawat, C. S., Flynn, W. F. Jr., Saddler, S., Hansraj, K. K., & Maynard, M. J. (1993). Long-term results of the total condylar knee arthroplasty: A 15-year survivorship study. *Clinical Orthopaedics and Related Research, 286*, 94–102.

Rand, J. A. (1991). Role of arthroscopy in osteoarthritis of the knee. *Arthroscopy, 7*(4), 358–363.

Rissanen, P., Seppo, A., Slatis, P., Sintonen, H., & Paavolainen, P. (1995). Health and quality of life before and after hip arthroplasty. *Journal of Arthroplasty, 10*, 169–175.

Ritter, M. A., Gandolf, V. S., & Holston, K. S. (1989). Continuous passive motion versus physical therapy in total knee replacements. *Clinical Orthopaedics and Related Research, 244*, 239.

Roach, J. A., Trembray, L. M., & Bowers, D. L. (1995). Preoperative assessment and education program implementation and outcomes. *Patient Education Counsel, 25*, 83–88.

Rudan, J. F., & Simurda, M. A. (1990). High tibial osteotomy: A prospective clinical and roentgenographic review. *Clinical Orthopaedics and Related Research, 255*, 251–256.

Rudan, J. F., & Simurda, M. A. (1991). Valgus high tibial osteotomy: A long-term follow-up study. *Clinical Orthopaedics and Related Research, 268*, 157–160.

Salter, R. B., Clements, N. D., & Ogilvie-Harris, D. (1982). The healing of articular tissues through continuous passive motion: Essence of the first 10 years of experimental investigations. *Journal of Bone and Joint Surgery, 64B*, 640.

Schumacher, H. R. (Ed.). (1993). *Primer on the rheumatic diseases*. Atlanta, GA: Arthritis Foundation.

Scott, R. J., & Huskisson, E. C. (1976). Graphic representation of pain. *Pain, 2*, 175–184.

Smeltzer, S. C., & Bare, B. G. (1992). *Brummer and Suddarth's textbook of medical-surgical nursing*. Philadelphia: Lippincott.

Spalding, T. J. W., Kiss, J., & Kyberd, P. (1994). Driver reaction times after total knee arthroplasty. *Journal of Bone and Joint Surgery, 76B*, 754–756.

Specchiulli, F., Laforgia, R., & Solarino, G. B. (1990). Tibial osteotomy in the treatment of varus osteoarthritic knee. *Italian Journal Orthopedic Traumatology, 16*(4), 507–514.

Steindler, A. (1955). *Kinesiology of the human body.* Springfield, IL: Charles C. Thomas.

Stern, S. H., Bowen, M. K., Insall, J. N., & Scuderi, G. R. (1990). Cemented total knee arthroplasty for gonarthrosis in patients 55 years old or younger. *Clinical Orthopaedics and Related Research, 260,* 124–129.

Stern, S. H., & Insall, J. N. (1992). Posterior stabilized prosthesis: Results after follow-up of nine to twelve years. *Journal of Bone and Joint Surgery, 74A,* 980–986.

Tinetti, M. E. (1986). Performance oriented assessment of mobility problems in elderly patients. *Journal of the American Gerontological Society, 34,* 119–125.

Tinetti, M. E., & Speechley, M. (1989). Prevention of falls among the elderly. *New England Journal of Medicine, 320,* 1055–1059.

Ververeli, P. A., Sutton, D. C., Hearn, S. L., & Booth, R. E. (1995). Continuous passive motion after total knee arthroplasty: Analysis of cost and benefit. *Clinical Orthopaedics and Related Research, 321,* 208–215.

Ward, E. S., & Jackson, N. W. (1992). Acid peptic disorders. In E. T. Herfindak, D. R. Gourley, & L. L. Hart (Eds.), *Clinical pharmacy and therapeutics* (pp. 393–398). Baltimore: Williams & Wilkins.

Ware, J., & Sherbourne, C. (1992). The MOS 36 item short form health survey (SF-36). *Medical Care, 30,* 473–483.

Windsor, R. E., Insall, J. N., Urs, W. K., Miller, D. V., & Brause, B. D. (1990). Two-stage reimplantation for the salvage of total knee arthroplasty complicated by infection: Further follow-up and refinement of indications. *Journal of Bone and Joint Surgery, 72A,* 272–278.

Yack, H. J., Collins, C. E., & Wheldon, T. J. (1993). Comparison of closed and open kinetic chain exercises in the anterior cruciate ligament-deficient knee. *American Journal of Sports Medicine, 21,* 49–54.

Yasuda, K., Majima, T., Tsuchida, T., & Kaneda, K. (1992). A 10 to 15-year follow-up observation of high tibial osteotomy in medial compartment osteoarthrosis. *Clinical Orthopaedics and Related Research, 282,* 186–195.

Appendix 1
Tinetti Gait and Balance Assessment Tool

Tinetti Assessment Tool _____ Date _____

Gait

1. Initiation of gait	Any hesitancy or multiple attempts	0	— — — — — —
	No hesitancy	1	— — — — —
2. Step length and height	A. RIGHT swing foot does not pass left stance foot with step	0	
	passes left stance foot	1	— — — — —
	right foot does not clear floor completely with step	0	
	right foot completely clears floor	1	— — — — —
	B. LEFT swing foot		
	does not pass right stance foot with step	0	
	passes right stance foot	1	— — — — —
	left foot does not clear floor completely with step	0	
	left foot completely clears floor	1	— — — — —
3. Step symmetry	Right & Left step length not equal	0	
	Right & Left step length are equal	1	— — — — —
4. Step continuity	Stopping or discontinuity between step	0	
	Steps appear continuous	1	— — — — —
5. Path	Marked deviation	0	
	Mild/Moderate deviation or uses walking aid	1	— — — — —
	Straight without walking aid	2	— — — — —
6. Trunk	Marked sway or uses walking aid	0	
	No sway but flexion of knees or back or spread arms out while walking	1	
	No sway, no flexion, no use of arms and no use of walking aid	2	— — — — —
7. Walking stance	Heels apart	0	
	Heels almost touching	1	— — — — —
Total			/12 /12 /12 /12 /12

Appendix 1 (cont.)

Tinetti Assessment Tool _____ Date _____

Balance

1. Sitting Balance	Leans, slides in chair	0	___ ___ ___ ___ ___
	Steady, Safe	1	___ ___ ___ ___ ___
2. Arises	Unable without help	0	
	Able, uses arms to help	1	___ ___ ___ ___ ___
	Able without using arms	2	___ ___ ___ ___ ___
3. Attempts to Arise	Unable without help	0	
	Able requires >1 attempt	1	___ ___ ___ ___ ___
	Able to arise, 1 attempt	2	___ ___ ___ ___ ___
4. Immediate Standing Balance	First 5 seconds		
	Unsteady (swaggers, moves feet, trunk sway)	0	
	Steady but uses walker or other support	1	___ ___ ___ ___ ___
	Steady without walker or other support	2	___ ___ ___ ___ ___
5. Standing Balance	Unsteady	0	
	Steady but wide stance (medial heels >4 inches apart, Uses cane or other support	1	___ ___ ___ ___ ___
	Narrow stance without support	2	___ ___ ___ ___ ___
6. Nudged (feet as close together as possible, examiner pushes lightly on subject's sternum with palm of hand 3 times	Begins to Fall	0	
	Staggers, grabs, catches self	1	___ ___ ___ ___ ___
	Steady	2	___ ___ ___ ___ ___
7. Eyes Closed	Unsteady	0	
	Steady	1	___ ___ ___ ___ ___
8. Turning 360 deg.	Discontinuous Steps	0	
	Continuous	1	___ ___ ___ ___ ___
	Unsteady (grabs, staggers)	0	
	Steady	1	___ ___ ___ ___ ___
9. Sitting down	Unsafe (misjudged distance falls into chair)	0	
	Uses arms or not a smooth motion	1	___ ___ ___ ___ ___
	Safe, smooth motion	2	
Balance score /16			/16 /16 /16 /16 /16

Appendix 2

The Western Ontario MacMaster Universities Osteoarthritis Index

Section A

The following questions concern the amount of **pain** you are currently experiencing due to arthritis in your hips, and/or knees. (Please mark your answer with an "X".)

QUESTION: How much pain do you have?

1. Walking on a flat surface.

NO PAIN |————————————————————| EXTREME PAIN

2. Going up or down stairs

NO PAIN |————————————————————| EXTREME PAIN

3. At night while in bed.

NO PAIN |————————————————————| EXTREME PAIN

4. Sitting or lying.

NO PAIN |————————————————————| EXTREME PAIN

5. Standing upright.

NO PAIN |————————————————————| EXTREME PAIN

Section B

The following questions concern the amount of joint stiffness (not pain) you are currently experiencing due to arthritis in your hips, and/or knees. Stiffness is a sensation of restriction or slowness in the ease with which you move your joints. (Please mark your answer with an "X".)

1. How severe is your stiffness after first awakening in the morning?

NO STIFFNESS |————————————————————| EXTREME STIFFNESS

2. How severe is your stiffness after sitting, lying or resting later in the day?

NO STIFFNESS |————————————————————| EXTREME STIFFNESS

Note. When this scale is reproduced for patients, the analog lines should be 10 cm. From "Validation study of the WOMAC: A health status instrument for measuring clinically important patient relevant outcomes to anti-rheumatic drug therapy in patients with osteoarthritis of the hip or knee," by N. Bellamy, W. W. Buchanan, C. H. Goldsmith, J. Campbell, and L. Stitt, 1988, *Journal of Rheumatology, 15*, pp. 1833–1840. Copyright 1988 by Allen Press. Reprinted with permission.

Appendix 2 (cont.)

Section C

The following questions concern your physical function. By this we mean your ability to move around and look after yourself. For each of the following activities, please indicate the degree of **difficulty** you are currently experiencing due to arthritis in your hips, and/or knees. (Please mark your answer with "X".)

QUESTION: What degree of difficulty do you have with:

1. Descending stairs.
   NO DIFFICULTY |————————————————| EXTREME DIFFICULTY

2. Ascending stairs.
   NO DIFFICULTY |————————————————| EXTREME DIFFICULTY

3. Rising from sitting.
   NO DIFFICULTY |————————————————| EXTREME DIFFICULTY

4. Standing.
   NO DIFFICULTY |————————————————| EXTREME DIFFICULTY

5. Bending to floor.
   NO DIFFICULTY |————————————————| EXTREME DIFFICULTY

6. Walking on flat.
   NO DIFFICULTY |————————————————| EXTREME DIFFICULTY

7. Getting in/out of car.
   NO DIFFICULTY |————————————————| EXTREME DIFFICULTY

8. Going shopping.
   NO DIFFICULTY |————————————————| EXTREME DIFFICULTY

9. Putting on socks/stockings.
   NO DIFFICULTY |————————————————| EXTREME DIFFICULTY

10. Rising from bed.
    NO DIFFICULTY |————————————————| EXTREME DIFFICULTY

11. Taking off socks/stockings.
    NO DIFFICULTY |————————————————| EXTREME DIFFICULTY

12. Lying in bed.
    NO DIFFICULTY |————————————————| EXTREME DIFFICULTY

Appendix 3

University of Pittsburgh—St. Margaret Hospital Mulitdisciplinary Documentation for Total Knee Surgery

UNIVERSITY *of* PITTSBURGH
MEDICAL CENTER
St. Margaret

**MULTIDISCIPLINARY DOCUMENTATION
TOTAL KNEE**

I. Pre-Admission (initial at left if complete)

Pre-operative Medical Record completed prior to	Video
surgery (H & P, Nsg. Assessment, CBC/diff	Review Surgical Procedure
PAC 9, U/A, EKG, surgical/anes. transfusion consents)	Pain Management Education
Blood Donation Completed #autologous	Unit Orientation
Direct_____	Post-operative Instruction
Donors_____	
None_____	
Social Service Card Sent	

Initials/Signature Section

II. Social/Home Status/Functional Status Pre-Admission

Home Status
☐ One Story
☐ Two Story
☐ Split Level
☐ Apartment
☐ PCBH
☐ ECF

Resides
☐ Alone
☐ Spouse
☐ Caretaker
☐ Family
  Members
☐ Other

Stairs
Outside #_____
  ☐ single ☐ double ☐ no rail
Inside #_____
  ☐ single ☐ double ☐ no rail
☐ No stairs/Doesn't use stairs

Occupation/Household Responsibilities/Comments:
☐ Cooking   ☐ Laundry
☐ Cleaning   ☐ Grocery Shopping

Comments: _____

Location of:
Bathroom ☐ 1st ☐ 2nd Floor
Bedroom   ☐ 1st ☐ 2nd Floor

Prior Community Services:
☐ Home Health ☐ Access ☐ Meals on Wheels
☐ Other _____

Ambulation
☐ Independent Without Device
☐ Independent With Device
_____
☐ Requires Assistance
☐ Non-Ambulatory
☐ Unknown

Transfers
☐ Independent
☐ Requires Assistance
☐ Total Dependence
☐ Unknown

Endurance
☐ Community Ambulator
☐ Household Ambulator
☐ N/A
☐ Unknown

Equipment Owned
☐ Standard/Wheeled/Platform Walker
☐ Straight/Quad Cane
☐ Wheelchair
☐ Axillary/Platform Crutches
☐ None/Unknown

Preliminary D/C Plans: Signature   Date

Physical Therapy Pre-op Evaluation

Comments: _____

Signature   Date

Occupational Therapy/ADL Pre-op Evaluation

Comments: _____

Signature   Date

MRL-304 (Rev. 8/96)

Note. From the University of Pittsburgh Medical Center—St. Margaret Hospital. Reprinted with permission.

Appendix 3 (cont.)

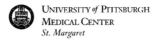

UNIVERSITY *of* PITTSBURGH
MEDICAL CENTER
St. Margaret

MULTIDISCIPLINARY DOCUMENTATION
TOTAL KNEE

DAY 1 DATE	Admission Day of Surgery			DAY 2 DATE	Post-op Day 1		
Medications	11-7	7-3	3-11	**Medications**	11-7	7-3	3-11
Pain Management Education				Pain Management Education			
Circle - Epidural, PCA, IM Injection				Circle - Epidural, PCA, IM Injection			
IV therapy per order				IV therapy per order			
Adequate Pain Relief				Adequate Pain Relief			
Prophylaxis/Medication Instruction				Prophylaxis/Medication Instruction			
				Blood transfusion if indicated			
				Nursing Assessment	11-7	7-3	3-11
				Alert & oriented x3			
Nursing Assessment	11-7	7-3	3-11	Neuro checks Q4° within normal limits			
Post-Op Nsg. Assess. form completed				Skin intact			
Alert & oriented x3				Knee Dsg. intact drainage may be present			
Neuro checks Q2° within normal limits				Drain intact			
Skin intact				Voiding s̄ problems via bedpan			
Knee Dsg. intact drainage may be present				Requiring intermittent catheterization			
Drain intact				Tolerating post-op lite or gen. diet			
Voiding s̄ problems via bedpan				Primary/Safety Standard of Care			
Foley				**Respiratory Assessment**	11-7	7-3	3-11
Requiring intermittent catheterization				Education Reinforced			
Tolerating CL or post-op lite				IS Q4° WA			
BS present				C & DB Q4°			
Primary/Safety Standard of Care				O2 _____ L as ordered			
				Respiration Unlabored			
				Activity	11-7	7-3	3-11
Respiratory Assessment	11-7	7-3	3-11	Begin Bed → Chair			
Respiratory Education				Pulsatile stockings			
IS Q2° WA				TEDS when OOB			
C & DB Q4°				Reinforce TKR Education			
O2 _____ L as ordered							
Respirations Unlabored							

PT Signature_____
☐ 1x/day ☐BID

TRANSFERS:
  sup ↔ sit ☐MAX ☐**MOD** ☐MIN ☐CS ☐⑤ ☐①
  sit ↔ stand ☐MAX ☐**MOD** ☐MIN ☐CS ☐⑤ ☐①
AMBULATION: ☐MAX ☐**MOD** ☐MIN ☐CS ☐⑤ ☐①
  Device ☐Walker ☐Crutches ☐Platform Walker ☐Parallel Bars
  Distance _____ feet WB status ☐WBAT ☐PWB ☐TDWB

HEP: QS, GS, AP, AROM, SLR, SAQ

Activity	11-7	7-3	3-11
Bedrest - turning side to side			
Pulsatile stockings			
TKR Education			
Immobilize as per protocol			

Documentational Instructions

- Initial all applicable items

- (/) slash - indicates non-applicable items

- (V) variable - abnormal findings - must document in nurses notes

Appendix 3 (cont.)

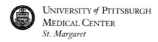

UNIVERSITY *of* PITTSBURGH
MEDICAL CENTER
St. Margaret

MULTIDISCIPLINARY DOCUMENTATION
TOTAL KNEE

DAY 3 DATE _____ Post-op Day 2 | **DAY 4** DATE _____ Post-op Day 3

Medications	11-7	7-3	3-11
Pain Management Instruction Reinforced			
Adequate Pain Relief			
Heparin Lock			
Prophylaxis/Medication Instruction			

Nursing Assessment	11-7	7-3	3-11
Alert & oriented x3			
Neuro checks Q8° within normal limits			
Skin intact			
Post-op Dsg. changed			
Drain to be removed today			
Voiding s̄ problems			
Diet as tolerated (DAT)			
Check for BM & document on graphic			
Primary/Safety Standard of Care			

Respiratory Assessment	11-7	7-3	3-11
Education Reinforced			
IS Q4° WA			
C & DB Q4°			
O₂ D/C			
Respirations unlabored			

Activity	11-7	7-3	3-11
Assist Amb. to BR / with device _____			
Pulsatile stockings			
TEDS/Remove BID			
Reinforce knee flexing with board			
Reinforce TKR Education			

PT Signature_____

☐ Ambulatory devices to room   ☐ Sliding board sent to Room

☐ 1x/day   ☐ BID
TRANSFERS:
  sup ↔ sit ☐ MAX   **☐ MOD**   ☐ MIN   ☐ CS   ☐ Ⓢ   ☐ Ⓘ
  sit ↔ stand ☐ MAX   ☐ MOD   **☐ MIN**   ☐ CS   ☐ Ⓢ   ☐ Ⓘ
AMBULATION: ☐ MAX   **☐ MOD**   ☐ MIN   ☐ CS   ☐ Ⓢ   ☐ Ⓘ
  Device   ☐ Walker   ☐ Crutches   ☐ Platform Walker
  Distance ☐ ≥ 25 feet or _____ feet   WB status ☐ WBAT   ☐ PWB   ☐ TDWB
HEP: QS, GS, AP, AROM, SLR, SAQ,
Knee ROM: Flexion _____   Extension _____

OT Signature_____
TRANSFERS:
  Chair: (w/c/std.)   ☐ Ⓘ   ☐ Ⓘ c̄ device   ☐ S   **☐ MIN**   ☐ MOD   ☐ MAX
  Bed: supine ↔ sit   ☐ Ⓘ   ☐ Ⓘ c̄ device   ☐ S   **☐ MIN**   ☐ MOD   ☐ MAX
    sit ↔ stand   ☐ Ⓘ   ☐ Ⓘ c̄ device   ☐ S   **☐ MIN**   ☐ MOD   ☐ MAX
  Toilet: ☐ Ⓘ   ☐ Ⓘ c̄ device   ☐ S   **☐ MIN**   ☐ MOD   ☐ MAX
  Bathing: ☐ Ⓘ   ☐ Ⓘ c̄ device   ☐ S   **☐ MIN**   ☐ MOD   ☐ MAX
  Dressing: ☐ Ⓘ   ☐ Ⓘ c̄ device   ☐ S   **☐ MIN**   ☐ MOD   ☐ MAX
☐ Review Education

Medications	11-7	7-3	3-11
Adequate Pain Relief			
Heparin Lock			

Nursing Assessment	11-7	7-3	3-11
Neuro checks q8° within normal limits			
Skin intact			
Incision Care Instruction			
Dressing change			
Voiding s̄ problems in BR			
Check for BM/Document			
DAT			
Primary/Safety Standard of Care			

Respiratory Assessment	11-7	7-3	3-11
IS prn			
Respirations unlabored			

Activity	11-7	7-3	3-11
Ambulates to BR with device _____			
TEDS/Remove BID			
D/C Pulsatile stockings			
Reinforce knee flexion with board			

PT Signature_____

☐ 1x/day   ☐ BID
TRANSFERS:
  sup ↔ sit ☐ MAX   ☐ MOD   **☐ MIN**   ☐ CS   ☐ Ⓢ   ☐ Ⓘ
  sit ↔ stand ☐ MAX   ☐ MOD   ☐ MIN   **☐ CS**   ☐ Ⓢ   ☐ Ⓘ
AMBULATION: ☐ MAX   ☐ MOD   **☐ MIN**   ☐ CS   ☐ Ⓢ   ☐ Ⓘ
  Device   ☐ Walker   ☐ Crutches   ☐ Platform Walker
  Distance ☐ ≥ 50 feet or _____ feet   WB status ☐ WBAT   ☐ PWB   ☐ TDWB
STAIRS: ☐ MAX   ☐ MOD   **☐ MIN**   ☐ CS   ☐ Ⓢ   ☐ Ⓘ
RAILS: ☐ 0   ☐ 1   ☐ 2   ☐ Cane   ☐ Crutches   ☐ None
HEP: ☐ Ⓘ   or ☐ _____
Knee ROM: Flexion _____   Extension _____

OT Signature_____
TRANSFERS:
  Chair: (w/c/std.)   ☐ Ⓘ   ☐ Ⓘ c̄ device   **☐ S**   ☐ MIN   ☐ MOD   ☐ MAX
  Bed: supine ↔ sit   ☐ Ⓘ   ☐ Ⓘ c̄ device   **☐ S**   ☐ MIN   ☐ MOD   ☐ MAX
    sit ↔ stand   ☐ Ⓘ   ☐ Ⓘ c̄ device   **☐ S**   ☐ MIN   ☐ MOD   ☐ MAX
  Toilet: ☐ Ⓘ   ☐ Ⓘ c̄ device   **☐ S**   ☐ MIN   ☐ MOD   ☐ MAX
  Tub/Shower: ☐ Ⓘ   ☐ Ⓘ c̄ device   **☐ S**   ☐ MIN   ☐ MOD   ☐ MAX
  Bathing: ☐ Ⓘ   ☐ Ⓘ c̄ device   **☐ S**   ☐ MIN   ☐ MOD   ☐ MAX
  Dressing: ☐ Ⓘ   ☐ Ⓘ c̄ device   **☐ S**   ☐ MIN   ☐ MOD   ☐ MAX
  Assess meal prep (pm)   ☐ Ⓘ   ☐ Ⓘ c̄ device   ☐ S   **☐ MIN**   ☐ MOD   ☐ MAX
☐ Review Education

Appendix 3 (cont.)

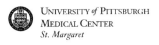

UNIVERSITY *of* PITTSBURGH
MEDICAL CENTER
St. Margaret

MULTIDISCIPLINARY DOCUMENTATION
TOTAL KNEE

DAY 5 DATE		Post-op Day 4	**DAY 6** DATE		Post-op Day 5

Medications	11-7	7-3	3-11	**Medications**	11-7	7-3	3-11
Adequate Pain Relief				Adequate Pain Relief			

Nursing Assessment	11-7	7-3	3-11	**Nursing Assessment**	11-7	7-3	3-11
Neuro checks q8° within normal limits				Neuro checks q8° within normal limits			
Skin intact				Skin intact			
Dressing change				Dressing change			
Voiding s̄ problems in BR				Voiding s̄ problem in BR			
Check for BM/Document				Elimination s̄ difficulty			
DAT				DAT			
Primary/Safety Standard of Care				Primary/Safety Standard of Care			

Activity	11-7	7-3	3-11	**Activity**	11-7	7-3	3-11
Amb. with device _____				Amb. with device _____			
TEDS/Remove BID				TEDS/Remove BID			
Knee flexion with board				Knee flexion with board			

PT Signature_____

☐ 1x/day ☐ BID
TRANSFERS:
    sup ↔ sit ☐ MAX ☐ MOD ☐ MIN ☐ CS ☐Ⓢ ☐①
    sit ↔ stand ☐ MAX ☐ MOD ☐ MIN ☐ CS ☐Ⓢ ☐①
AMBULATION: ☐ MAX ☐ MOD ☐ MIN ☐ CS ☐Ⓢ ☐①
    Device ☐ Walker ☐ Crutches ☐ Platform Walker
    Distance ☐ ≥ 75 feet or _____ feet WB status ☐ WBAT ☐ PWB ☐ TDWB
STAIRS: ☐ MAX ☐ MOD ☐ MIN ☐ CS ☐Ⓢ ☐①
RAILS: ☐ 0 ☐ 1 ☐ 2 ☐ Cane ☐ Crutches ☐ None
HEP: ☐① or ☐ _____

Knee ROM: Flexion _____ Extension _____

OT Signature_____
TRANSFERS:
Chair: (w/c/std.)	☐①	☐① c̄ device	☐ S	☐ MIN	☐ MOD	☐ MAX
Bed: supine ↔ sit	☐①	☐① c̄ device	☐ S	☐ MIN	☐ MOD	☐ MAX
sit ↔ stand	☐①	☐① c̄ device	☐ S	☐ MIN	☐ MOD	☐ MAX
Toilet:	☐①	☐① c̄ device	☐ S	☐ MIN	☐ MOD	☐ MAX
Tub/Shower:	☐①	☐① c̄ device	☐ S	☐ MIN	☐ MOD	☐ MAX
Bathing:	☐①	☐① c̄ device	☐ S	☐ MIN	☐ MOD	☐ MAX
Dressing:	☐①	☐① c̄ device	☐ S	☐ MIN	☐ MOD	☐ MAX
Meal prep (pm)	☐①	☐① c̄ device	☐ S	☐ MIN	☐ MOD	☐ MAX
☐ Review Education

Initials/Signature Section

PT Signature_____

☐ 1x/day ☐ BID
TRANSFERS:
    sup ↔ sit ☐ MAX ☐ MOD ☐ MIN ☐ CS ☐Ⓢ ☐①
    sit ↔ stand ☐ MAX ☐ MOD ☐ MIN ☐ CS ☐Ⓢ ☐①
AMBULATION: ☐ MAX ☐ MOD ☐ MIN ☐ CS ☐Ⓢ ☐①
    Device ☐ Walker ☐ Crutches ☐ Platform Walker
    Distance ☐ ≥ 100 feet or _____ feet WB status ☐ WBAT ☐ PWB ☐ TDWB
STAIRS: ☐ MAX ☐ MOD ☐ MIN ☐ CS ☐Ⓢ ☐①
RAILS: ☐ 0 ☐ 1 ☐ 2 ☐ Cane ☐ Crutches ☐ None
HEP: ☐① or ☐ _____

Knee ROM: Flexion _____ Extension _____

OT Signature_____
TRANSFERS:
Chair: (w/c/std.)	☐①	☐① c̄ device	☐ S	☐ MIN	☐ MOD	☐ MAX
Bed: supine ↔ sit	☐①	☐① c̄ device	☐ S	☐ MIN	☐ MOD	☐ MAX
sit ↔ stand	☐①	☐① c̄ device	☐ S	☐ MIN	☐ MOD	☐ MAX
Toilet:	☐①	☐① c̄ device	☐ S	☐ MIN	☐ MOD	☐ MAX
Tub/Shower:	☐①	☐① c̄ device	☐ S	☐ MIN	☐ MOD	☐ MAX
Bathing:	☐①	☐① c̄ device	☐ S	☐ MIN	☐ MOD	☐ MAX
Dressing:	☐①	☐① c̄ device	☐ S	☐ MIN	☐ MOD	☐ MAX
Meal prep (pm)	☐①	☐① c̄ device	☐ S	☐ MIN	☐ MOD	☐ MAX
☐ Review Education

Initials/Signature Section

Appendix 3 (cont.)

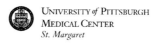

UNIVERSITY *of* PITTSBURGH
MEDICAL CENTER
St. Margaret

**MULTIDISCIPLINARY DOCUMENTATION
TOTAL KNEE**

Discharge Instructions

Occupational Therapy

Transfers	Goal Achieved	Goal Not Achieved	ADL's	Goal Achieved	Goal Not Achieved
Chair	☐	☐	Dressing	☐	☐
Bed	☐	☐	Bathing/Hygiene	☐	☐
Toilet	☐	☐	Meal Prep(pm)	☐	☐
Tub/Shower	☐	☐			
Review Car	☐	☐			

Patient demonstrated ability to incorporate patient education and safety into ADL's.   ☐ Achieved   ☐ Not Achieved

_____ out of _____ goals achieved. The following goals were not achieved secondary to:

_____

_____

Comments: _____

_____

EQUIPMENT: ☐ Long sponge   ☐ Dressing stick   ☐ Sock device   ☐ Elastic Laces   ☐ Long shoehorn   ☐ Elevated toilet   ☐ Shower stool
☐ Leg lifter   ☐ Reacher   ☐ Other_____

Signature: _____

Physical Therapy

GOALS: Achieved   Not Achieved

[ ] 1. I SUPV CS MIN MOD MAX transfers supine < >sit   [ ]   [ ]

[ ] 2. I SUPV CS MIN MOD MAX transfers sit < > stand   [ ]   [ ]

[ ] 3. I SUPV CS MIN MOD MAX stairs with ☐ 0 ☐ 1 ☐ 2 rails and/or devices: [ ]   [ ]
       Device: ☐ cane   ☐ crutches   ☐ platform crutch   ☐ walker   ☐ other _____
       ☐ stairs not required ☐ 1 step only

[ ] 4. I SUPV CS MIN MOD MAX ambulation with device   [ ]   [ ]
       Device: ☐ cane   ☐ crutches   ☐ platform walker   ☐ walker   ☐ other _____

[ ] 5. Ambulation _____ feet or greater   ☐ NWB   ☐ TDWB   ☐ PWB   ☐ WBAT   [ ]   [ ]

[ ] 6. ⓘ with written home exercise program   [ ]   [ ]

[ ] 7. Patient demonstrates understanding of precautions.   [ ]   [ ]

[ ] 8. _____   [ ]   [ ]

[ ] 9. _____   [ ]   [ ]

[ ] 10. _____   [ ]   [ ]

Other Physical Findings: _____

_____

A: _____ out of _____ goals achieved. The following goals were not achieved 2° to: _____

_____

_____

Comments: _____

_____

P: Pt D/C to: ☐ Home   ☐ PCH   ☐ ECF   ☐ SMMH Rehab   ☐ SMMH TCU   ☐ Other_____
     Follow-up:

Signature _____

Appendix 4

The Hospital for Special Surgery
Knee Service
Knee Rating Sheet

Name _____ HSS # _____ Preoperative date _____

		LEFT						RIGHT					
PAIN (30 points)	Score	pre	6 mo	1 yr	2 yr	3 yr	4 yr	pre	6 mo	1 yr	2 yr	3 yr	4 yr
Walking: none	15												
mild	10												
moderate	5												
severe	0												
At rest: none	15												
mild	10												
moderate	5												
severe	0												
FUNCTION (22 points) Walk:													
walking and standing unlimited	12												
5-10 blocks, standing > 30 min	10												
1-5 blocks, standing 15-30 min	8												
walk < 1 block	4												
cannot walk	0												
Stairs: normal	5												
with support	2												
Transfer: normal	5												
with support	2												
ROM (18 points) each 8″ = 1 point													
MUSCLE STRENGTH (10 points)													
cannot break quadriceps	10												
can break quadriceps	8												
can move through arc of motion	4												
cannot move through arc of motion	0												
FLEXION DEFORMITY (10 points)													
none	10												
5″-10″	8												
10″-20″	5												
>20″	0												
INSTABILITY (10 points)													
none	10												
0″-5″	8												
6″-15″	5												
>15	0												
TOTAL													
SUBTRACTIONS:													
one cane	1												
one crutch	2												
two crutches	3												
extension lag of 5″	2												
10″	3												
15″	5												
Deformity (5″ = 1 point) varus													
valgus													
TOTAL SUBTRACTIONS													
KNEE SCORE													

Note. From The Hospital for Special Surgery, New York, NY. Reprinted with permission.

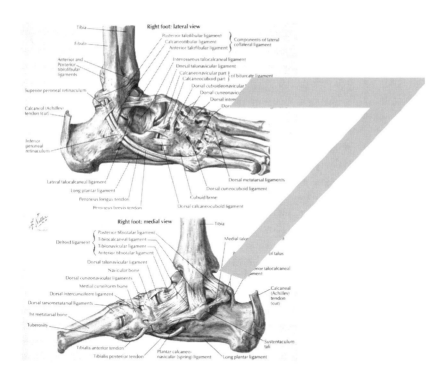

Right foot: lateral view

Tibia
Fibula
Anterior and Posterior tibiofibular ligaments
Superior peroneal retinaculum
Calcaneal (Achilles) tendon (cut)
Inferior peroneal retinaculum
Lateral talocalcaneal ligament
Long plantar ligament
Peroneus longus tendon
Peroneus brevis tendon

Posterior talofibular ligament
Calcaneofibular ligament } Components of lateral
Anterior talofibular ligament } collateral ligament
Interosseous talocalcaneal ligament
Dorsal talonavicular ligament
Calcaneonavicular part } of bifurcate ligament
Calcaneocuboid part }
Dorsal cuboideonavicular
Dorsal cuneonavicular
Dorsal inter
Dor

Dorsal metatarsal ligaments
Dorsal cuneocuboid ligament
Cuboid bone
Dorsal calcaneocuboid ligament

Right foot: medial view

Deltoid ligament {
Posterior tibiotalar ligament
Tibiocalcaneal ligament
Tibionavicular ligament
Anterior tibiotalar ligament
Dorsal talonavicular ligament
Navicular bone
Dorsal cuneonavicular ligaments
Medial cuneiform bone
Dorsal intercuneiform ligament
Dorsal tarsometatarsal ligaments
1st metatarsal bone
Tuberosity
Tibialis anterior tendon
Tibialis posterior tendon

Tibia
Medial talo
of talus
ior talocalcaneal
ament
Calcaneal (Achilles) tendon (cut)
Sustentaculum tali
Plantar calcaneo-navicular (spring) ligament
Long plantar ligament

RHEUMATOID ARTHRITIS IN THE FOOT AND ANKLE: SURGERY AND REHABILITATION

Andrea Cracchiolo, III, MD, Dennis Janisse, CPed, and Victoria Gall, MEd, PT

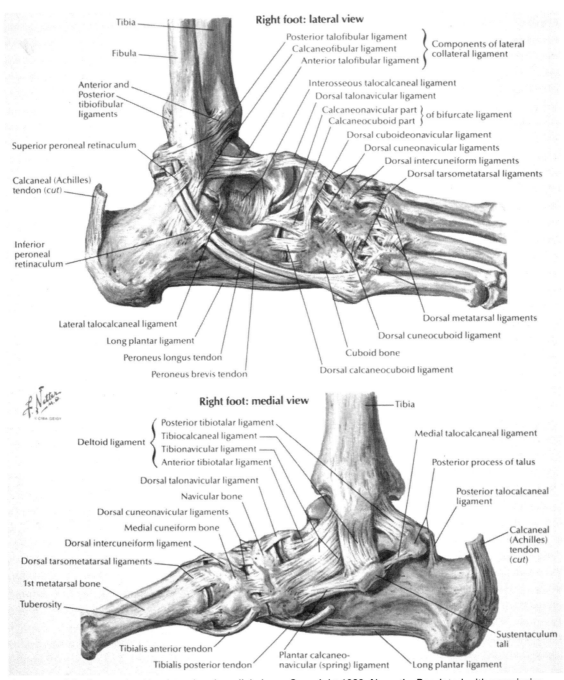

Right foot: lateral view

Tibia

Fibula

Anterior and Posterior tibiofibular ligaments

Superior peroneal retinaculum

Calcaneal (Achilles) tendon (*cut*)

Inferior peroneal retinaculum

Posterior talofibular ligament
Calcaneofibular ligament
Anterior talofibular ligament
} Components of lateral collateral ligament

Interosseous talocalcaneal ligament
Dorsal talonavicular ligament
Calcaneonavicular part
Calcaneocuboid part
} of bifurcate ligament
Dorsal cuboideonavicular ligament
Dorsal cuneonavicular ligaments
Dorsal intercuneiform ligaments
Dorsal tarsometatarsal ligaments

Dorsal metatarsal ligaments

Dorsal cuneocuboid ligament

Cuboid bone

Dorsal calcaneocuboid ligament

Lateral talocalcaneal ligament
Long plantar ligament
Peroneus longus tendon
Peroneus brevis tendon

Right foot: medial view

Tibia

Deltoid ligament {
Posterior tibiotalar ligament
Tibiocalcaneal ligament
Tibionavicular ligament
Anterior tibiotalar ligament

Medial talocalcaneal ligament

Posterior process of talus

Posterior talocalcaneal ligament

Dorsal talonavicular ligament
Navicular bone
Dorsal cuneonavicular ligaments
Medial cuneiform bone
Dorsal intercuneiform ligament
Dorsal tarsometatarsal ligaments
1st metatarsal bone
Tuberosity

Calcaneal (Achilles) tendon (*cut*)

Sustentaculum tali

Tibialis anterior tendon
Tibialis posterior tendon
Plantar calcaneonavicular (spring) ligament
Long plantar ligament

Anatomy of the foot and ankle—lateral and medial views. Copyright 1989. Novartis. Reprinted with permission from the *Atlas of Human Anatomy*, illustrated by Frank H. Netter, MD. All rights reserved.

When the feet hurt, just about everything else can hurt. Dysfunction in the ankle and foot area can transfer pain to the knees, hip, and back. Rheumatoid arthritis (RA) can affect all the joints in the foot and ankle, and the problems are often a combination of mechanical and inflammatory stressors. If activity levels are lessened because of the pain, then flexibility, strength, and cardiovascular fitness will decrease. Therapy and prescription shoes both play a role in conservative management to prevent or lessen the need for surgery and postoperatively to improve gait and to maximize comfort and function. Pincus and Callahan (1992) have shown that decreased function in RA is associated with increased mortality. This further supports the importance of keeping patients ambulatory. This chapter reviews the pathology seen in the foot and ankle of persons with RA, discusses conservative management in detail, and then describes common surgical interventions and postoperative rehabilitation.

RA of the Foot and Ankle

RA is a systemic disease that involves the foot as frequently as it does the hand. During the course of the disease, the forefoot is involved in up to 89% of patients with RA, the hindfoot in up to 67%, and the ankle joint in only about 9% of patients (Benson & Johnson, 1971). Because there are many synovial-lined joints within the foot, active rheumatoid disease can produce widespread foot pain. Joint swelling can probably be best seen in the forefoot in the metatarsophalangeal (MTP) joints. Swelling can likewise be seen surrounding the tendon sheaths across the dorsum of the ankle, along the posterior tibialis tendon, and occasionally along the peroneal tendons. Swelling of the hindfoot is best seen at the talonavicular joint medially and over the sinus tarsi laterally.

The classic findings of RA in the forefoot include hallux valgus with intra-articular degeneration of the MTP joints (Figure 1). Synovitis of the MTP joints usually occurs early in the progression of the disease (Spiegel & Spiegel, 1982). The toes drift laterally with dorsal subluxation or dislocation. The kinematics of push off during gait cause stretch of the plantar capsule and supporting ligaments. As this occurs, the metatarsal heads are directed more plantarward, the toes develop a clawtoe (hammer toe) deformity at the interphalangeal joints, and the weight-bearing plantar fat pad is drawn further forward and loses its normal location underneath the metatarsal heads. Patients report that this feels like "walking on marbles." The metatarsal heads are frequently destroyed by a combination of the synovitis and disturbed anatomy. Large bursae with overlying calluses are frequent under the middle metatarsal heads and at times under the hallux. Web space pathology, usually an intermetatarsal bursa in the third web space, gives neuroma-like symptoms as an early sign of forefoot involvement, and this in fact may be an early sign of RA (Awerbuch, Shephard, & Vernon-Roberts, 1982; Dedrich, McCune, & Smith, 1990; Shephard, 1975).

Pathology of the hindfoot is more subtle, can progress rapidly, and frequently affects the forefoot. Synovitis of the hindfoot joints and subsequent loss of articular cartilage and erosion of the talonavicular and subtalar joints lead to a characteristic valgus deformity of the hindfoot. The talonavicular joint becomes unstable with the head of the talus drifting medially and plantarward (Elbar,

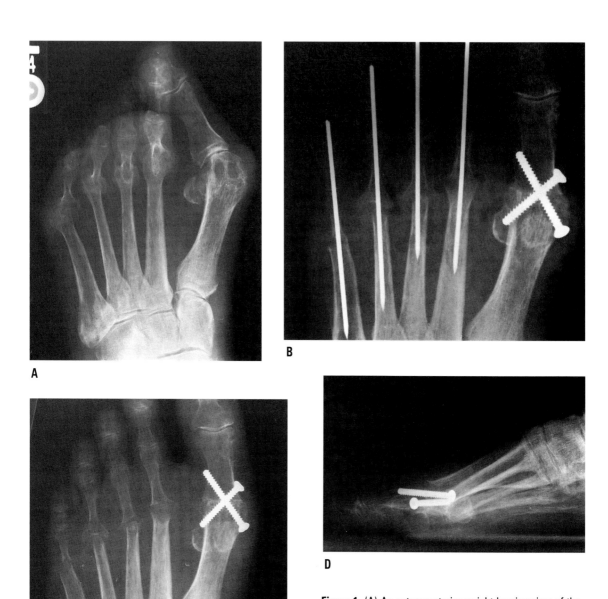

Figure 1. (A) An anteroposterior weight-bearing view of the left foot. A woman (54 years of age) with RA for 18 years with typical forefoot deformities—severe hallux valgus erosion and dislocation of the lateral four metatarsal phalangeal joints. Excessive cysts are noted in the first metatarsal head. Because of the bone quality and the excessive deformity, an arthrodesis of the hallux metatarsal phalangeal joint was advised. (B) A postoperative radiograph showing two 3.5-mm screws placed across the first metatarsophalangeal joint to assist in the arthrodesis. The lateral four metatarsophalangeal joints have undergone a plantar plate arthroplasty. The 0.062-in. Kirschner wires will hold the corrected alignment of the lateral four toes. The wires are usually removed between the 3rd and 4th week postoperatively. (C) One year postoperatively, the hallux metatarsophalangeal joint has successfully fused. The screws are not painful for the patient and will remain in place. The lateral four rays are well aligned. (D) A lateral weight-bearing view of the left foot showing correct alignment for the hallux fusion in approximately 30° of extension from the first metatarsal. The patient had an excellent result with long-term maintenance of correction and no pain. She was able to wear athletic shoes and some styles of noncorrective shoes comfortably.

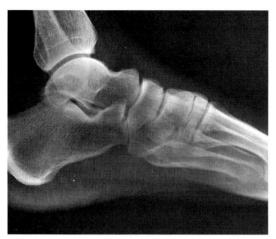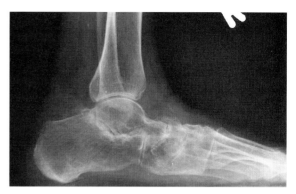

Figure 2. (A, left) Lateral non–weight-bearing radiograph of the right foot of a patient with RA for 2 years. Note increased thickening of the plantar heel pad. (B, right) Weight-bearing lateral radiograph of the right foot taken 3 years later (5 years after the onset of disease). Note the rapid progression of involvement of all of the hindfoot joints (e.g., subtalar, talonavicular, and calcaneocuboid joints). The talus has drifted into plantar flexion, and the arch has fallen. This patient had severe hindfoot pain. Fortunately, the ankle joint was spared at this time. The patient required a triple arthrodesis.

Thomas, Weinfeld, & Potter, 1976). The remainder of the midfoot and forefoot drifts into abduction, and the longitudinal arch flattens (Figure 2). The calcaneus may abut against the distal fibula, thus producing pain at the lateral malleolus (Cracchiolo, Pearson, Kitaoka, & Grace, 1990). The posterior tibial tendon may rupture (Downey, Simkin, Mack, Richardson, Kilcayne, & Hansen, 1988) or, if intact, may not function effectively as the medial stabilizer of the hindfoot because of the altered hindfoot mechanics. Only 8% of patients with disease for less than 5 years had moderate to severe hindfoot deformities (Spiegel & Spiegel, 1982). However, in patients with disease for more than 5 years, 25% had abnormal hindfoot valgus on weight bearing (Spiegel & Spiegel, 1982).

Ankle pathology gives far fewer symptoms, and when patients complain of ankle pain, most are actually experiencing hindfoot pain in the subtalar joint. Ankle instability can result from erosions of the dome of the talus and ligament instability such that a valgus deformity may result from pathology within the tibiotalar joint rather than the hindfoot. It is essential to make this distinction between hindfoot and ankle pathology, but ankle joint pathology is less frequent (Cracchiolo, Cimino, & Lian, 1992).

Evaluation

Radiographic Imaging

A set of plain radiographs is typically obtained. This includes weight-bearing anteroposterior and lateral views of the foot. Additionally, a weight-bearing anteroposterior view of the ankles is important, especially if there is any ankle or hindfoot pathology. There are no general indications for the use of computerized axial tomography scans and magnetic resonance imaging techniques because radiographic films are usually sufficient.

Function

Most health status indexes and functional evaluations ask questions about walking, but none focuses specifically on the foot and ankle. The Foot Function Index (Appendix 1) was developed at a Chicago's Veterans Hospital and is a self-evaluation of pain and disability with a visual analog format (Budiman-Mak, Conrad, & Roach, 1991). (*Note.* On this scale, the scoring line must be 10 cm. Patients are given one point for every centimeter, zero points for no centimeters, and 10 points for all the time.)

The patient's gait, at the least, should be observed with and without shoes and assisted devices on flat surfaces at varying speeds. Greater detail can be obtained from videotaping the activity. Motion analysis in a gait laboratory can be extremely helpful in complex cases.

Conservative Management: Footwear

The most important aspect of nonoperative care is proper footwear in patients with RA (Cracchiolo, 1979, 1982). Often, the first time a patient with arthritis is prescribed footwear is after surgery. This is unfortunate because proper footwear early in the disease course can accommodate many foot conditions and improves comfort, joint support, and ease of walking and may often delay or even prevent the need for surgery. Usually, a shoe must be selected or modified to fit the patient's deformity. Shoes do not correct deformities; rather, they accommodate the deformities and thus reduce pain. This improves ambulation and balance and reduces fatigue associated with inefficient walking or pain. Because the forefoot is the most common area of symptoms and pathology, a shoe with a wider and deeper toe box is important for patients with RA. Podiatrists can play an important role in conservative management of toe deformities, skin breakdown, and callosities through evaluation and prescription of accommodative footwear and othoses (Roth, 1986).

A pedorthist is a board-certified (CPed) specialist in providing and fabricating prescription footwear, including shoes, modifications, and orthoses (Janisse, 1995a). A physical therapist is in a key position in the health care system to provide a comprehensive evaluation of foot–ankle mechanics and gait and to make recommendations for exercise as well as foot orthoses and proper footwear. Physical therapists who specialize in treating the foot can additionally fabricate simple orthoses and make shoe modifications.

The role of the occupational therapy practitioner varies. In Canada and other western countries, the occupational therapy practitioner is often trained in fitting and customizing foot orthoses. In some facilities, they may make custom sandals. Occupational therapy practitioners can make custom assistive devices to facilitate donning and doffing of shoes and stockings as well as training patients in adaptive dressing techniques and use of commercial devices.

Although there are mail-order companies that make custom orthoses, it is better for the person with RA to have a local contact because often the insert needs modification, and this can better be done in person. Because custom orthoses are not reimbursable items through most insurance companies, it is essential that the patient receives the appropriate device and has it modified according to symptoms. This often requires many revisions by the orthotic technician.

For patients with polyarticular disease such as RA, the ability to don and remove stockings and shoes is an important consideration. There are many assistive devices to accomplish this task, including long-handled shoe horns, dressing sticks, adaptive Velcro® closures, elastic shoe laces, and sock and stocking donners. For a current listing of adaptive dressing aids, one can search the Abledata database on the Internet (www.Abledata.com). Guidelines for proper foot care are listed in Appendix 2.

Internal Shoe Modifications

Metatarsal pads. These are one of the most common shoe modifications. They shift weight-bearing pressure proximal to the MTP heads, rather than directly on the heads, and reduce stress to the MTP joints. These pads are recommended as a method for protecting the MTP joints early in the course of the disease. When used by themselves, they should be placed with the apex of the pad just proximal to the area of maximum tenderness or callus formation, usually between the second and third metatarsal heads. For RA foot involvement, it is more common to have the pads built into the orthosis.

Heel cushions or cups. Sponge cushions with a hole cut to relieve pressure over heel spurs are helpful for many patients, but they may require a shoe with extra depth (Clark, 1996). Prefabricated rubber or plastic heel cups can help reduce pain associated with Achilles enthesitis, plantar fasciitis, or subcalcaneal spurs. Heel cups mold the soft tissues to provide greater protection between the tender point and the shoe during weight bearing (Clark, 1996). These cups can be provided by occupational therapy and physical therapy departments. The health care provider should provide advice on exercise, weight reduction, and joint protection with an ambulatory device when needed. Most soft-tissue problems are caused by overuse, and when there is a predisposing mechanical problem, the incidence and reoccurrence rate increases. Gel-type heel cushions are effective for treatment of plantar fasciitis and heel spurs. A pair should be worn even if the problem is unilateral because the thickness of the material may affect leg length and gait.

Foam shoe liners. There are many commercially available products that will help the simpler problems. They include liners for cushioning and distributing weight-bearing pressure over the sole rather than bony prominences. Some come with metatarsal pads or wedges built into them.

External Shoe Modifications

The outside of the shoe can be modified in various ways to accommodate virtually any foot shape, deformity, or other foot condition associated with arthritis. The most commonly prescribed external shoe modifications include rocker soles, extended steel shanks, stabilization, cushion heels, wedges, and extensions.

Rocker sole. As its name suggests, the basic function of a rocker sole is to literally "rock" the foot from heel-strike to toe-off without bending the shoe. The actual shape of a rocker sole varies according to the desired effect or purpose of the rocker sole and the patient's specific foot problems. In general, the biomechanical effects of a rocker sole are to compensate for lost motion in the foot or ankle related to pain, deformity, or stiffness, which results in an overall improvement in gait and relieves pressure on some area of the plantar surface.

Many athletic shoes, usually labeled as running or walking shoes, are made with a mild rocker sole (see Figure 3A). This generic rocker sole, which provides some metatarsal relief and gait assistance, is often adequate for many patients. However, a rocker sole can be custom-made to relieve more specific or more severe problem areas. A system of six basic rocker-sole types, including the variation of the degree and location of rocker angles, is illustrated in Figure 3. When prescribing a rocker sole, it is essential that the physician clearly specify the desired effect or purpose of the rocker sole. A certified pedorthist is trained to know which type of rocker sole will best achieve that purpose. The pedorthist will take measurements, obtain floor reaction imprints, and provide follow-up care to make sure that the rocker sole is performing properly for the patient.

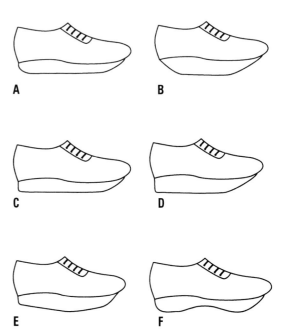

Figure 3. Six types of rocker soles. (A) Mild, with a mild rocker angle at both heel and toe. (B) Heel to toe, with a more severe rocker angle at heel and toe. (C) Toe only, with a mild rocker angle only at the toe. (D) Severe angle, with a more severe rocker angle at the toe only. (E) Negative heel, with a mild rocker angle at the toe and a negative heel. (F) Double, a mild rocker sole with a section of the sole removed in the midfoot area, thereby giving the appearance of two rocker soles (one at the hindfoot and one at the forefoot).

Extended steel shank. An extended steel shank is a strip of spring steel that is inserted between the layers of the sole and extends from the heel to the toe of the shoe. It is most commonly used in combination with a rocker sole and will often make the rocker sole more effective. An extended steel shank can prevent the shoe from bending, limit toe and midfoot motion, aid propulsion on toe-off, and strengthen the entire shoe and sole.

Stabilization. This type of external shoe modification involves the addition of material to the medial or lateral portion of the shoe to stabilize some part of the foot. A flare is an extension to the heel or heel and sole of the shoe (Figure 4). Flares can be medial or lateral, and their purpose is to stabilize the hindfoot, midfoot, or forefoot. For example, a medial heel flare might be used to support a valgus heel deformity. A stabilizer is an extension added to the side of the shoe, including both the sole and upper. Made from rigid foam or crepe, a stabilizer provides more stabilization than a flare and is used for more severe medial or lateral instability of the hindfoot or midfoot.

Solid ankle cushion heel (SACH). A SACH consists of a wedge of shock-absorbing material that is added at the heel of the shoe. Its purpose is to provide a maximum amount of shock absorption under the heel, for example, in the case of a loss of fatty tissue in the heel area.

Wedge. A wedge of sole material is sometimes added medially or laterally to the heel of the shoe or to both the heel and sole (Figure 5). It can be inserted between the upper and the sole or added directly to the bottom of the shoe to redirect the weight-bearing position of the foot. A wedge is useful in stabilizing a flexible deformity in a corrected position or in accommodating a

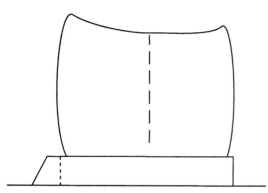

Figure 4. Medial flare.

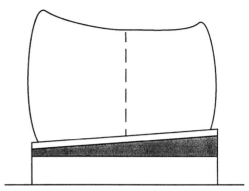

Figure 5. Lateral wedge.

fixed deformity (by essentially bringing the ground to the foot). A medial wedge is indicated in cases of extreme pronation, whereas a lateral wedge can be used for ankle instability or a varus heel deformity.

Extension. An extension consists of material added to the sole of a shoe to increase the height or thickness of the sole. Extensions may be added to the heel area only or to the entire sole and heel. When an extension is added only to the heel area of the sole, its purpose is usually to accommodate a fixed deformity or to relieve hindfoot pressure. A complete heel and sole extension is used to eliminate a leg-length discrepancy. Depending on its height, the extension is generally made of crepe, leather, or rigid foam, and the larger extensions are generally used in conjunction with a rocker sole. Extensions can be used with a wide variety of shoes, including athletic footwear and dress shoes, and can be covered with matching upper material to achieve cosmetically pleasing results.

Custom-Made Foot Orthoses

A custom-made foot orthosis (CFO) is a special insert made from a model of the patient's foot. CFOs include the shell that is the top layer of material in contact with the bottom of the foot and the posting, which is the material that fills in the space between the shell and the shoe. A CFO may have additional layers between the shell and the posting and can be further customized by adding small amounts of additional materials to specific areas, such as a sponge rubber metatarsal pad or viscoelastic polymer under the heel.

Because CFOs are made from a model of the patient's foot, they are said to be in "total contact" with the foot. The combination of total contact with the use of appropriate materials means that CFOs can fulfill the objectives listed in Table 1 in the following ways:

1. CFOs relieve pressure from sensitive or painful areas by evenly distributing pressure over the entire plantar surface.
2. CFOs reduce shock through the use of shock-absorbing materials and reduce shear because the total contact minimizes horizontal foot movement.
3. CFOs accommodate and support deformities. Fixed or rigid deformities can be accommodated with the use of soft materials in the shell. Flexible deformities can be supported with the use of more rigid, supportive materials in the CFO posting.

Table 1. Objectives for the Pedorthic Care of RA of the Foot and Ankle

Although each patient's needs are different, and prescription footwear must be individualized, there are certain basic objectives:

1. *Relieve pressure* from sensitive or painful areas such as metatarsal heads, nodules, or bony prominences.

2. *Reduce shock and shear.* In addition to relieving specific high-pressure areas, prescription footwear can be helpful in decreasing the overall amount of vertical pressure, or shock, on the foot. A reduction in the horizontal movement of the foot within the shoe, or shear, can likewise be achieved. Shock and shear reduction are particularly important for patients with RA because of their sensitive skin, loss of fatty tissue, and because the joints can be inflamed, painful, and stiff, thus making them more sensitive to shock and shear forces.

3. *Accommodate and support deformities.* Fixed or rigid deformities can be accommodated with the use of soft materials in shoes and orthoses, and certain shoe modifications can help replace lost joint motion. Prescription footwear can be helpful in providing needed support, correction, and pain relief for more flexible deformities.

4. *Control or limit motion of joints.* Limiting the motion of certain foot and ankle joints through the use of prescription footwear can often decrease inflammation, relieve pain, and result in a more stable and functional foot.

4. CFOs control or limit joint motion. Limiting the motion of certain foot and ankle joints can be achieved through the use of supportive materials in the CFO.

Depending on which of these objectives is primary, a given CFO can be described as either accommodative or functional. An accommodative CFO is designed primarily to accommodate a rigid foot or one that is particularly at risk, and a functional CFO is designed to control a more flexible foot by providing support or stability. CFOs used for persons with arthritis tend to be accommodative, but most CFOs will have both functional and accommodative properties and are, of course, customized to meet each patient's needs.

Although there are many materials currently used to fabricate CFOs, they can be divided into three basic types (Janisse, 1995b).

1. *Soft.* Cross-linked polyethylene foams are the most common soft materials currently used for persons with arthritis. They are made by many manufacturers and are rapidly being developed and improved. They are generally moldable with the application of heat (250°–300°) and come in various densities. Their function is accommodative. Studies show, however, that they decrease in thickness rather quickly, a phenomenon referred to as "bottoming out."

2. *Semiflexible.* Leather and cork fall into this category. Many of the cork materials are now combined with plastic compounds to make them moldable when heated. Semiflexible materials are somewhat accommodative but provide more functional support than the soft type and do not bottom out as quickly.

3. *Rigid.* Acrylic plastics, thermoplastic polymers, and graphite combinations are considered rigid materials. They are moldable at high temperatures and are primarily functional in nature. They are the most durable and most supportive of the three types.

Most CFOs are made of a combination of materials, with the softer materials in the shell and more rigid materials in the posting. Some manufacturers are now making multiple-layer materials, which eliminate the time-consuming process of manually combining CFO layers.

In-Depth Shoes

The basic shoe used in the vast majority of arthritis footwear prescriptions is the in-depth shoe. It is designed with an additional 1/4 to 3/8-in. depth throughout the shoe, which provides enough room for a generic insole or a CFO and allows extra volume for the foot inside the shoe. In-depth shoes can accommodate common arthritis foot deformities including prominent metatarsal heads, hallux valgus, hammer toes, nodules, and bony prominences.

In-depth shoes usually come in a basic oxford style but are increasingly available as both athletic and dress shoes. They are available in a wide range of shapes and sizes for both men and women and can be used for all but the most severely deformed foot. They are made with various upper materials, including cowhide and deerskin, and some have uppers that can be heat molded to a patient's foot shape. In-depth shoes are generally lightweight, have shock-absorbing soles and strong heel counters, and come with a rocker sole to assist with walking.

Custom-Made Shoes

A custom-made shoe is constructed from a cast or model of the patient's foot and is needed only in rare cases when extremely severe deformities are present that prohibit the use of an in-depth shoe, even with extensive modifications. Modified in-depth shoes are generally preferred over custom-made shoes because they can be provided in less time, at a lower cost, and have a better appearance.

Preoperative Considerations

Gait Training and Modifications

Preoperative gait training is more common than ever because many foot surgeries are day procedures. Most ankle procedures require hospitalization. Often, the patient will already use ambulatory devices because of pain. It is essential for the surgeon to consider the patient's upper-extremity joint status when discussing the postoperative course. Platform crutches may be indicated for patients with elbow, wrist, or hand problems; however, they are heavy and difficult to use, so practice is necessary.

The patient should be alerted to the fact that crutch use, particularly when it is for a non–weight-bearing gait pattern or for long lengths of time, may increase shoulder and neck symptoms. Activity modifications and adjustments to the home and work environment should be considered before the day of surgery. More assistance from others may be needed. (Postoperative interventions of the physical therapist will be discussed later in this chapter.)

Surgical Staging

Lower-extremity surgery is usually preferable, if possible, before upper-extremity surgery because of the need for ambulatory devices that place a great amount of pressure on the shoulders, elbows, and wrists. If the hips and knees are destroyed, they will usually require surgical correction. The forefoot is overwhelmingly more often painful than the hindfoot or the ankle. Surgery in the forefoot is 8 times more common than hindfoot surgery, and it usually precedes surgery of the hindfoot or ankle.

The Effect of Medication on the Surgical Procedure

One of the most important preoperative considerations should be the patient's current medications. Patients taking 10 mg of prednisone daily, and certainly greater than 15 mg, are at high risk for failure of primary wound healing (Cracchiolo et al., 1992) and developing sepsis. Methotrexate delays wound healing and, if possible, should be discontinued about 1 week before surgery and for 2 weeks postoperatively.

Tourniquet Placement

Thigh-high tourniquet control is recommended for foot surgery in RA. Usually there are gross deformities of the toes, and a tourniquet applied above the ankle tends to bind the tendons, which in turn interferes with the soft-tissue correction of deformities. Vasculitis or peripheral vascular disease are contraindications for the use of a tourniquet.

Surgery and Rehabilitation for the Forefoot

Arthroplasty

Historically, the destroyed MTP joint was simply excised without reconstruction in patients with RA. This operation was performed for many years, and almost all conceivable varieties of excisional arthroplasty, through various dorsal and plantar incisions, have been described (Barton, 1973; Cracchiolo, 1988; Craxford, Stevens, & Park, 1982; Faithful & Savill, 1971; Gainor, Epstein, Henstorf, & Olson, 1988; Hassalo, Wilkens, Toomey, Darges, & Hansen, 1987; Hughes, Grace, Clark, & Klenerman, 1991; Mann & Thompson, 1984; McGarvey & Johnson, 1988; Stockey et al., 1989; Vahvanen, Pirainen, & Kettunen, 1980; Watson, 1974). The excision of both the metatarsal head and the base of the proximal phalanx was popularized by Clayton (1982) who, after extensive clinical experience, advocated that if one or two joints were relatively spared by the disease, they should be excised so that all MTP joints are included in the forefoot operation. Clayton (1982) emphasized that the postoperative results of these procedures on the rheumatoid forefoot will gradually deteriorate if the patient is followed long enough. Rheumatoid disease is frequently progressive, and if deformities increase in the hindfoot and midfoot joints, then forefoot deformities may recur. One should avoid the indiscriminate resection of bone as the only method of correcting the forefoot deformity; it is as important to realign the soft-tissue structures as it is to resect the bone.

McGarvey and Johnson (1988) reviewed 20 series involving more than 1,730 ft in which the RA forefoot was reconstructed. Eight surgeons performed multiple procedures and were able to conclude only that forefoot surgery in RA was beneficial, but the benefit may not be long lasting (Amuso, Wissinger, Margolis, Eisenbeis, & Stolzer, 1971; Craxford et al., 1982; Hassalo et al., 1987). Most series report satisfactory results in up to 85% of patients (the range is 55% to 100%) and failures of less than 10% (Amuso et al., 1971; Clayton, 1982; Craxford et al., 1982; Faithful & Savill, 1971; Hughes et al., 1991; Kates, Kessel, & Kay, 1967; Mann & Thompson, 1984; Morgan, Henke, Bailey, & Kaufer, 1985; Newman & Fitton, 1983). Vahvanen et al., 1980; Watson, 1974). Factors associated with unfavorable results include:

- inadequate bony resection (Faithful & Savill, 1971; Vahvanen et al., 1980; Watson, 1974),
- recurrent hallux valgus (Watson, 1974),
- wound problems (Faithful & Savill, 1971; Lipscomb, Benson, & Sones, 1972; Newman & Fitton, 1983),
- disease progression (Hassalo et al., 1987), and
- neurovascular problems (Kates et al., 1967; McGarvey & Johnson, 1988).

Surgery for the Lateral Four Metatarsophalangeal Joints

The metatarsal head is most frequently resected because it is usually grossly destroyed and pushed plantarward by the dorsally dislocated toes. The surgeon must then decide whether to resect the base of the proximal phalanx. This may not be necessary in all patients. Excision of the proximal one third usually results in a loss of control of the toe, and thus the toe may become floppy. Excising the base of the proximal phalanx should only be done in conjunction with syndactylization (i.e., webbing the toes by suturing portions of the skin of toes 2 to 3 and toes 4 to 5). It is a most useful procedure to correct severely deformed toes or when revision forefoot operations are performed. There are three basic surgical procedures for correcting deformity of the lateral four MTP joints: plantar plate arthroplasty, excisional arthroplasty, and a platar approach.

Plantar plate arthroplasty. This procedure is a distinct improvement over excisional arthroplasty (Clayton, 1982). The lateral four MTP joints are approached in sequence (Cracchiolo, 1984).

If the joints are severely dislocated, it is better to release the extensor tendons, ligaments, and capsule of all four joints before attempting to expose the metatarsal heads. A small amount of the base of the proximal phalanx is resected, thus freeing the plantar plate, which is placed over the resected end of the metatarsal and transfixed with a 0.062-in. Kirschner wire (Figure 6). The wire stabilizes the alignment of the ray. Some patients have a "stiff type" of rheumatoid disease, and the wires can be removed at about 2 to 3 weeks. Those with a "loose type" of disease should have the wires in place for about 5 weeks.

Excisional arthroplasty. Excisional arthroplasty can be performed through a web space incision that allows excision of the head of the metatarsal as well as the base of the proximal phalanx (Daly & Johnson, 1982). The incision is then sutured so that a syndactylization is performed, which stabilizes the adjacent toes.

A plantar approach. A plantar approach to the dislocated MTP joints can be performed when only the MTP heads are to be resected (Kates et al., 1967). Excision of some of the redundant skin helps to keep the fat pad

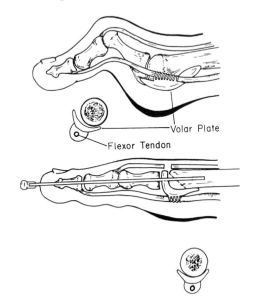

Figure 6. A schematic diagram of the volar (plantar) plate arthroplasty. The metatarsal head is resected obliquely, and the volar plate, if present, is dissected and placed between the resected ends of the metatarsophalangeal joint. This centralizes the flexor tendon.

properly repositioned. This incision should be used when the dorsal skin is poor and when the patient may have had previous operations with inappropriately placed dorsal scars.

Surgery for the First MTP Joint in RA

Occasionally, the hallux MTP joint may be spared. However, if there is major synovitis, an arthrotomy should be performed through a longitudinal incision, and a synovectomy should be carried out. If there is a great hallux valgus deformity with good joint space, this must be corrected to accommodate the more normal realignment of the lateral four toes. In most cases, there is major joint destruction with a severe valgus deformity. There are two surgical options, either of which should be performed after correction of the lateral four MTP joints: arthrodesis and implant arthroplasty.

Arthrodesis. There are many techniques used to surgically fuse the first MTP joint. It may be best to create two flat surfaces so that there is some intrinsic stability to the arthrodesis site (Figures 1B and 1C) (Cracchiolo, 1984). The lateral rays will be shorter after all or part of the MTP joints have been excised; therefore, it is important to resect sufficient amounts of the metatarsal head and the base of the proximal phalanx so that the first ray will not be overly long. The final position of the hallux is important. Because of a lateral drift of the toes with time, it may be best to fuse the hallux in 20° to 25° of valgus. In addition, about 15° of dorsiflexion as measured from the floor, or about 30° as measured from the first metatarsal, is adequate (see Figure 1D). There should be no rotation of the toe, and the toenail should point directly dorsally. The hallux should not protrude more than about 1 cm beyond the second toe at the end of the procedure. Internal fixation is accomplished with various techniques. Multiple 0.062-in. Kirschner wires, either threaded or plain, have been used. Two 3.5-mm cortical screws placed as lag screws can be used if the quality of bone is good and if the medial flare of the proximal phalanx can be salvaged (see Figures 1A–1D). Recently, a 5- or 6-hole, one-quarter tubular plate fixed with 3.5-mm cortical screws has been used dorsally to hold the bony surfaces together until arthrodesis occurs (Cracchiolo, 1990). The plate must be bent to allow the proper angle of dorsiflexion. Unfortunately, the dorsal position of the plate allows it only to act as a neutralizing force so that the internal fixation may be suboptimal. All three of these methods share the advantage of not crossing the interphalangeal joint.

Implant arthroplasty of the hallux MTP joint. This is possible with a double-stem implant manufactured of a high-performance silicon elastomer (Cracchiolo, Swanson, & Swanson, 1981). The addition of a titanium grommet (sleeve) to protect the implant from rough bone ends appears to make the implant more stable, reduce radiolucency around the stems, and reduce fracture of the stems (Sebold & Cracchiolo, 1996; Swanson et al., 1991). Use of an implant will restore a more normal forefoot alignment and maintain some hallux motion (Figure 7). An ideal candidate for an implant arthroplasty is a patient with RA who has a subluxed or dislocated MTP joint with adequate bone stock and intact soft tissues and without evidence of sepsis or vascular insufficiency. Implants should only be used in a destroyed hallux MTP joint, which is usually the case in RA. Implants give the surgeon an alternative to performing an arthrodesis. They can be most helpful as a salvage procedure for patients with an unsatisfactory result after excision of the hallux MTP joint. Two long-term follow-up series indicate excellent outcomes in selected patients (Cracchiolo et al., 1981; Moeckel, Sculco, Alexiades, Dossick, & Inglis, 1992).

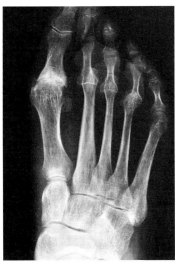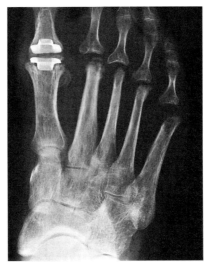

Figure 7. (A) An anteroposterior weight-bearing radiograph of the right foot of a woman with RA for 12 years. All of her joints are destroyed, and toes 2, 3, and 4 are dislocated at the metatarsophalangeal joint. Toe 5 is subluxated and painful. There are no major changes clinically or radiographically in the midfoot or hindfoot. Because of an acceptable alignment of the first ray and adequate bone stock, a double-stemmed silicone implant was advised. (B) Postoperative views at 1 year showing the double-stemmed silicone implant protected by titanium grommets. The lateral four rays were corrected with the plantar plate arthroplasty described earlier. This patient had a good long-term result and was able to wear some fashionable shoes with no pain.

Postoperative Management of Forefoot Surgery

The combination of good wound closure and a sterile compression dressing allows minimal wound hematoma. This is particularly important for procedures that do not require hospital admission and will not have frequent postoperative checks. All patients are encouraged to keep the leg elevated when sitting, even after ambulation has begun. They should be reminded that proper elevation requires that the torso is lower than the foot. Supporting the posterior knee and lower leg will lessen knee discomfort. The pillows should be placed parallel (under the knee and calf), not perpendicular to the knee. Merely sitting up with the knee and foot extended can increase back symptoms as well as knee pain.

Weight-bearing status and motion will be restricted, and specific guidelines must be written by the surgeon. Either a postoperative wooden shoe, a short leg cast, or a prefabricated walking cast is issued, depending on the surgery and the stability required.

A postoperative shoe is routine after a MTP fusion, but a cast may be needed when the patient is either osteoporotic or has difficulty with weight-bearing guidelines, which will last for at least 6 weeks (Alexander, 1994). When the wire extends beyond the toes, the patient should be cautioned to observe the foot when climbing stairs to avoid hitting or catching the wires on the riser. For MTP osteotomies, a cast may be changed to a postoperative shoe at 10 days, and the patient may return to normal footwear at 3 to 4 weeks, at which time exercises are started (Johnson, 1994). A postoperative shoe is most often given after Silastic™ implantation and is used for 4 to 6 weeks.

Crutches are most often given after these procedures, although a cane may be allowed if the guidelines indicate "weight bearing as tolerated." Most patients are hesitant to weight bear either because of the pain or because of the loss of sensation from slow resolution of the anesthetic. The practitioner or nurse must be prepared to teach a non–weight-bearing gait so that the patient is safe to be discharged. There are patients who have no pain, and they must be warned to obey the precautions because the foot will likely become more painful as the medication wears off and as activity progresses.

Therapy after multiple MTP procedures usually begins on postoperative day 1 or 2 depending on the swelling. Therapy consists of bed mobility, transfers, and progression to short-distance gait training. Gait will either be non-weight bearing or partial weight bearing (Saltman, 1996). The purpose of wooden postoperative shoes is to prevent forefoot motion. The bulky dressing holds the foot in slight dorsiflexion, which increases weight bearing force on the heel, thus making ambulation in the shoe more difficult for persons with limited ankle motion. A sturdy shoe should be worn on the nonoperative foot, preferably one with some height (1/2 in. to 3/4 in.), which will help during the swing phase of the operated leg. Knee and ankle ROM is encouraged within the confines of the bandage. Short, frequent walks are encouraged, and a nonreciprocal stair pattern is taught. Bilateral foot procedures make stair climbing difficult, particularly when the knees have limited motion. In these cases, it is easier and safer to descend the stairs sideways. The feet should be elevated between walking sessions. At the 4 to 6-week postoperative visit, most patients will be progressed to weight bearing as tolerated and will be allowed to wear regular shoes as long as they have adequate room for the reconstructed forefoot weight-bearing, motion, and footwear guidelines.

Surgical Correction and Rehabilitation of the Hindfoot

Tenosynovectomy

Hindfoot pathology most frequently involves the talonavicular and the talocalcaneal (subtalar) joints. The most important soft-tissue involvement is synovitis about the tendon sheath of the posterior tibialis, flexor digitorum longus, and flexor hallucis longus tendon (Cracchiolo, 1982; Russotti, Johnson, & Cass, 1988). Should nonoperative treatment fail to control this synovitis, the tendons should be released from their sheaths and the excess synovium resected. This procedure could prevent rupture of the posterior tibialis tendon, which has been described in rheumatoid patients (Michelson, Easley, Wigley, & Hellman, 1995). A patient is usually placed in a cast for 7 to 10 days, at which time strengthening exercise are begun, and the support is slowly discontinued. A medial wedge may be recommended for 6 months.

If a tendon is repaired or a transfer operation is performed, then the patient is casted for 6 weeks and progressed to a shoe with a medial heel and sole wedge. Physical therapy is indicated to mobilize the foot and strengthen the transferred muscles after the cast has been removed.

Arthrodesis

Stabilization of the rheumatoid hindfoot includes fusion of the subtalar (talocalcaneal) joint and the joints between these bones and the midtarsal bones. This surgery is frequently necessary and should be performed early before the development of severe hindfoot valgus deformity (Friscia, 1996). Some patients will only have destruction of the talonavicular joint with localized symptoms (Figure 8). Early arthrodesis of that joint has been advocated (Elbar, et al., 1976), and it is most

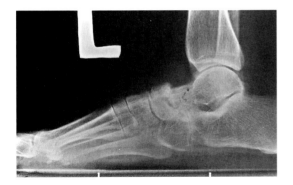 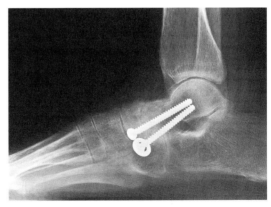

Figure 8. (A) The lateral weight-bearing radiograph of the left foot of a physician (44 years of age) with RA for 10 years. The talonavicular joint is completely destroyed, but the other joints of the hindfoot and midfoot as well as the ankle are relatively spared. (B) This patient is an ideal candidate for an isolated talonavicular joint fusion. This was performed with two 4.5-mm cortical screws placed as lag screws. She was in a cast for 4 weeks (non-weight bearing) and in a walking cast for 4 weeks. Postoperatively, her pain resolved completely, and she was able to continue work as a physician. The screws were not painful and have not as yet been removed. No physical therapy was required.

unusual for these patients to require additional hindfoot fusions. Such patients may, of course, represent a limited population whose other joints may have been spared anyway.

The ultimate aim of a successful hindfoot arthrodesis is to relieve hindfoot pain and to have the foot in a plantigrade position with the metatarsals level when the hindfoot is corrected to approximately 7° of valgus. The operative technique selected depends on the type of deformity. Various possibilities exist include:

- a hindfoot with no evidence of malalignment, which is rare;
- a hindfoot with a major valgus deformity, by far the most common pathology and more difficult to treat; and
- a varus malalignment usually associated with some cavus deformity, more commonly seen in juvenile rheumatoid arthritis.

A lateral weight-bearing radiograph of the foot (see Figure 8A) is most helpful in determining the angle of the talus to the first metatarsal bone. The talus normally should be aligned directly with the first metatarsal. In a severe valgus deformity, the talus will rotate medially and plantarward, and patients will have an angle of 15° or more between the two bones. An anteroposterior weight-bearing view of the ankle is essential. There may be a valgus deformity at the tibiotalar joint, and it is critical to know this preoperatively. A lateral view of the foot helps to evaluate tibiotalar arthritis, the degree of joint changes in the talonavicular and calcaneocuboid joints, and any forefoot pathology.

An arthrodesis of hindfoot joints (triple arthrodesis) is accomplished by removing the articular surfaces and roughening the underlying subchondral bone. Internal fixation is required using a 6.5-mm cancellous bone screw across the subtalar joint (about 65 mm long), one 4.5-mm screw from the navicular into the talus (about 50 mm long; a 6.5-mm screw may fracture the navicular tuberosity), and a single screw across the calcaneocuboid joint (about 35 mm long). The calcaneocuboid joint can be easily fixed with a powered staple gun that fires thin titanium staples across the joint.

Subtalar Bone Grafting

Two basic types of bone graft procedures can be performed to stabilize the subtalar joint. A dowel of bone from the ilium can be placed into a prepared dowel hole across the posterior facet of the joint (Cracchiolo, 1988; Cracchiolo et al., 1990), or the joint can be excised and filled with autogenous cancellous bone (King, Watkins, & Samuelson, 1980). A large-diameter threaded Steinmann pin can be used to stabilize the arthrodesis site. It is placed from the talus into the calcaneus to avoid any solid portion of the graft. The pin is left protruding through the skin and is removed in 4 to 6 weeks. Alternatively, a cancellous bone screw can be used for internal fixation.

Hindfoot Stabilization in Patients With Major Valgus Deformities

It is essential to correct the valgus deformity and not attempt to perform an arthrodesis, which would leave the patient with his or her original hindfoot deformity. Most deformities can usually be corrected by exposing the joints and by freeing the joint surfaces. It is occasionally necessary with a fixed valgus deformity to remove some of the head of the talus to be able to correct the overall foot deformity. In a severe valgus deformity, correction usually leaves a gap across the posterior facet of the subtalar joint, and this gap must be filled with bone. The hindfoot should not be overcorrected if there is a major forefoot deformity as well. There usually is enough residual midfoot motion so that the forefoot can compensate even when a severely deformed hindfoot is corrected. However, it may be necessary to do an arthrodesis on the hindfoot in 10° to 12° of valgus to maintain a plantigrade forefoot.

Postoperative Management of Hindfoot Surgery

Hindfoot procedures require hospital admission, and the anesthesia can be spinal or general. The foot is elevated for at least 24 hr before a cast is applied. The patient is instructed in a non–weight-bearing gait pattern. If the patient is having a difficult time remaining non-weight bearing, then a 1/2- to 3/4-in. tapered lift can be applied to the heel and sole of the weight-bearing shoe. This will facilitate clearing the casted leg during the swing phase, and it will lessen the need to hold the knee in as much flexion. At approximately 6 weeks, the patient will progress to partial weight bearing either in a Fiberglas cast or a removable walking cast and will continue wearing it until there is no pain with full weight bearing. The patient will progress to regular footwear with good longitudinal support or to prescriptive footwear. At this time, radiographs usually will not show a solid arthrodesis. Supports should continue until the patient is pain free, is not limping, and has good strength. The average time of immobilization and protected gait is 12 weeks.

After a triple arthrodesis, patients with RA usually report excellent pain relief. This appears to be related to achieving a solid fusion, no matter which technique is used (Cracchiolo, 1990; Feiwell & Cracchiolo, 1994; Figgie, O'Malley, Ranawat, Inglis, & Sculco, 1993). The rehabilitation for this procedure is similar to subtalar fusions; however, the length of immobilization will depend on patient age and surgical fixation. If an iliac bone graft is used, ambulation progress may be a little slower because of donor site pain. There may be some initial discomfort with sitting.

Many activities of daily living will have to be modified and be done in a sitting position. Information on cast covers for bathing should be given to all patients, and problem situations should be discussed with the physical therapist or occupational therapy practitioner. Endurance may be a problem because of the increased energy expenditure needed to walk with a device and with weight-bearing restrictions. An upper-extremity ROM and strengthening program should be encouraged.

Surgery and Rehabilitation of the Ankle Joint

Synovectomy

Persistent synovitis of the ankle resistant to conservative treatment may be a consideration for a synovectomy. A thorough lavage and debridement of the ankle with an arthroscopic technique may give great pain relief while retaining ankle joint motion. Open synovectomy of the ankle is another option.

A partial weight-bearing gait is necessary to rest the joint and allow healing. A removable walking cast may be helpful in relieving pain. A walking aid should be used to eliminate limping, which puts more stress on the joint. Ice and elevation are recommended.

Arthrodesis

The only reliable procedure to treat a painful destroyed ankle in RA continues to be ankle arthrodesis (Cracchiolo, 1992). This is usually done by way of subtalar arthrodesis because these patients may have involvement of other hindfoot and forefoot joints or lower-extremity joints. Many operations have been described for ankle arthrodesis, and although they are different, there are several common features that place the various techniques into groups:

- compression arthrodesis with an external fixator is used as an adjunct to many arthrodesis techniques,
- the fibula is used as a strut or spike graft, and
- the tibia is used as a donor site, such as with a sliding graft into the joint.

Internal fixation with the use of a plate and screws or rigid screw fixation has been reported; however, this may be insufficient fixation if moderate to severe osteoporosis is present (Cracchiolo, 1992; Morgan et al., 1985). A recent review of ankle fusions in patients with RA that use either internal fixation or compression arthrodesis with an external fixator yielded a fusion rate of 80%. Most of the failures were complicated by infection. The average time to fusion was 18 weeks.

The final position of the foot as it relates to the leg is an important factor in ankle fusions. The neutral position for arthrodesis appears to give the best overall results (Cracchiolo, Cimino, & Lian, 1992). If there has been a previous triple arthrodesis, or if the hindfoot is stiff, then it may be best to place the foot in about 5° of dorsiflexion because this may make it easier for the patient to get out of chairs. The talus should be covered by the tibial surface as posteriorly as possible so that the foot will not protrude because a long anterior lever arm will impede gait. The foot should be in 10° to 15° of external rotation in relation to the long axis of the leg. If the hindfoot is stiff or has been fused previously, the overall position of the foot must be plantigrade with the heel in valgus.

It is occasionally necessary to perform both an ankle and subtalar joint arthrodesis simultaneously (Figure 9). It is rarely necessary to include the transverse tarsal joints (pan-talar arthrodesis).

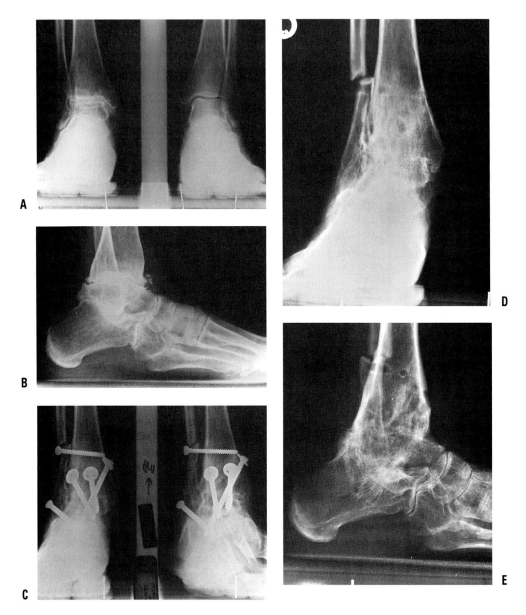

Figure 9. (A) An anterior weight-bearing radiograph of both ankles of a woman (47 years of age) with severe RA for 15 years. Her right ankle joint shows complete loss of the articular space. This joint was painful and would not permit the patient to walk outside of her home. She had already undergone bilateral total knee replacement and ipsilateral total hip replacement. (B) A lateral weight-bearing radiograph of same patient's right foot and ankle, which shows destruction of the ankle joint and narrowing of the subtalar joint. The patient also had pain on both the medial and lateral sides of the hindfoot indicating subtalar joint involvement. Fortunately, the talona-vicular and calcaneocuboid joints have been spared. (C) An anteroposterior and oblique weight-bearing radiograph of the patient's right ankle, approximately 18 months after arthrodesis. Both the subtalar joint and the tibiotalor joint have been fused with cancellous bone screws and the fibula as an onlay graft. (D) An anteroposterior weight-bearing radiograph of the patient's right ankle at 2 years after the operation. The screws were irritating the patient and giving some localized pain, and they were removed as an outpatient proce-dure. The ankle is solidly fused. (E) A lateral weight-bearing radiograph of the patient's right ankle and hindfoot, which shows a solid ankle and a solid subtalar fusion after removal of the screws. The patient is pain free and is able to walk well, grocery shop, and care for her family members.

These can be demanding surgical techniques, and the surgeon should have considerable experience with such cases or enlist assistance from a colleague with such experience.

The postoperative weight-bearing status for an ankle fusion is similar to subtalar fusions. The patient may benefit from either a commercially available or custom device to help raise the leg in and out of bed. When the fusion is solid, adaptations to the shoe may be needed to smooth out gait and to accommodate for a possible leg-length discrepancy.

Total Ankle Arthroplasty

Total ankle arthroplasty (TAA) is being performed by only a few orthopedic surgeons attempting to determine whether implants placed without cement may indeed result in good long-term arthroplasty. Cemented implants were commonly performed in the late 1970s and early 1980s, and most of them inevitably failed, so the procedure was abandoned for many years (Kitaoka & Johnson, 1996). Certainly, if there is adequate bone stock, it would be preferable to have a painless ankle that could have some motion in dorsiflexion and plantar flexion. However, failure of such an implant would require an ankle arthrodesis, which would be more difficult to perform after removing the implant. Thus, there is hesitation by many surgeons to again attempt to perform a TAA.

Postoperatively, regaining motion is not a problem and usually is not emphasized. After good wound healing, at least 10° to 15° dorsiflexion and 20° to 30° plantar flexion should be expected. Current protocols either call for the application of a short leg cast on POD 2 when drainage has ceased or for the use of a posterior splint. Percentage of weight bearing is dependent on fixation (Figgie, Unger, Inglis, Kraay, & Figgie, 1991).

Often patients, because of the systemic nature of their disease, must use platform crutches that are heavier and clumsier. Generally, they remain partially weight bearing for 4 to 6 weeks, at which time active motion is allowed. An ambulation aid should be continued as long as the gait is antalgic.

Postoperative Footwear

Immediately after surgery, the presence of swelling, edema, or bulky dressings may necessitate the use of some type of postoperative shoe before a regular in-depth or custom-made shoe can be worn.

- *Postoperative shoe.* This shoe can accommodate extreme swelling and the bulkiest dressings with a wide forefoot opening and Velcro® straps or lace closures. The uppers are made of canvas or nylon mesh, and most include a rigid sole to allow the patient to walk while limiting joint motion. It is the style of choice for all forefoot and midfoot surgeries.

- *Heat-moldable healing shoe.* This is used whenever a soft, flexible, accommodative healing shoe is needed; this closed-toe, extra-wide shoe is made from a nylon-covered moldable polyethylene foam and can be molded directly to the patient's foot.

- *Controlled ankle motion device.* For the patient who can be mobile but must maintain a fixed ankle position or limited ankle motion, the controlled ankle motion walker can provide the necessary stability and support while allowing a comfortable, natural gait pattern. This appliance is essentially a postoperative shoe to which medial–lateral uprights and a posterior Achilles plate have been added. The foot and ankle are held in place with wide Velcro® straps, and the ankle joint may be held in a fixed position or allowed to move within a limited ROM (up to 45°).

Although the basic objectives of prescription footwear will not change after surgery, there may be changes in the foot that must be accommodated. These include lost motion after fusion; change in the size or shape of the foot; restored, but possibly still limited, joint motion; and sensitive or vulnerable areas. Postoperatively, the objectives of prescription footwear are accomplished as follows:

- *Relieve pressure from sensitive or painful areas.* In addition to relieving pressure from a painful surgical site, new sensitive areas may be created by surgery. For example, after a metatarsal resection or hallux valgus correction, the remaining metatarsal heads will have increased weight bearing. A CFO and an appropriate rocker sole can help even out plantar pressure and prevent additional problems from this resulting transfer in weight bearing.

- *Reduce shock and shear.* After any type of fusion, the foot may lose some of its shock-absorbing ability; therefore, additional shock absorption must be provided, usually by a CFO, or, in the case of the heel area, with a SACH. It is important to minimize shear for any resulting sensitivity at the surgical site.

- *Accommodate and support deformities.* Fixed or rigid deformities after fusion can be accommodated with the use of soft materials in shoes and orthoses, and a rocker sole can help replace lost joint motion. If surgery results in a more flexible foot, for example, after arthroplasty of one or more metatarsal heads, a more functional CFO can be used to provide support.

- *Control or limit motion of joints.* Limiting motion of certain joints may become necessary after surgery. For example, after a triple arthrodesis, inversion and eversion ability is lost. A flare or stabilizer can help limit this motion. A heel extension may be needed depending on the resulting position of the fused foot.

Summary

Physical examination of the foot and ankle and evaluation of ambulation should be routine in patients with RA. Although surgery can reduce pain and increase function, early attention and preventive measures such as proper shoe selection, use of an orthosis, and podiatric care can help to alleviate the biomechanical stress on other joints, which in turn can help the patient remain active and ambulatory.

References

Alexander, I. J. (1994). Hallux interphalangeal fusion. In K. A. Johnson (Ed.), *Master techniques in orthopedics: The foot and ankle* (pp. 21–30). New York: Raven Press.

Amuso, S. J., Wissinger, H. A., Margolis, H. M., Eisenbeis, C. H. Jr., & Stolzer, B. L. (1971). Metatarsal head resection in the treatment of rheumatoid arthritis. *Clinical Orthopaedics and Related Research, 74*, 94–100.

Awerbuch, M. D., Shephard, E., & Vernon-Roberts, B. (1982). Morton's metatarsalgia due to intermetatarsophalangeal bursitis as an early manifestation of rheumatoid arthritis. *Clinical Orthopaedics and Related Research, 167*, 214–221.

Barton, N. J. (1973). Arthroplasty of the forefoot in rheumatoid arthritis. *Journal of Bone and Joint Surgery, 55B*, 126–133.

Benson, G. M., & Johnson, E. W. (1971). *Management of the foot in rheumatoid arthritis. Orthopedic Clinics of North America, 2*, 733–744.

Budiman-Mak, E., Conrad, K. J., & Roach, K. E. (1991). The foot functional index. *Journal of Clinical Epidemiology, 44*, 561–570.

Clark, B. M. (1996). Foot management and ambulatory aids. In S. T. Wegener & B. L. Belza (Eds.), *Clinical care in the rheumatic diseases* (pp. 95–101). Atlanta, GA: American College of Rheumatology.

Clayton, M. L. (1982). Evolution of surgery of the forefoot in rheumatoid arthritis. *Journal of Bone and Joint Surgery, 64B*, 640.

Cracchiolo, A. (1979). The use of shoes to treat foot disorders. *Orthopedic Review, 8*, 73.

Cracchiolo, A. (1982). Management of the arthritic forefoot. *Foot and Ankle, 3*, 17–23.

Cracchiolo, A. (1984). Surgery for rheumatoid disease: AAOS course lecture. *Mosby Times Mirror, 33*, 386.

Cracchiolo, A. (1988). Rheumatoid arthritis of the foot and ankle. In J. Gould (Ed.), *The foot book* (pp. 239–267). Baltimore: Williams & Wilkins.

Cracchiolo, A. (1990). Surgical arthrodesis techniques for foot and ankle pathology. *AAOS Instrumental Course Series, 39*, 49–63.

Cracchiolo, A., Cimino, W. R., & Lian, G. (1992). Arthrodesis of the ankle in patients who have rheumatoid arthritis. *Journal of Bone and Joint Surgery, 74A*, 903–909.

Cracchiolo, A., Pearson, S., Kitaoka, H. B., & Grace, D. (1990). Hindfoot arthrodesis in adults utilizing a dowel graft technique. *Clinical Orthopaedics and Related Research, 257*, 193–203.

Cracchiolo, A., Swanson, A., & Swanson, G. D. (1981). The arthritis great toe metatarsophalangeal joint: A review of flexible silicone implant arthroplasty from two medical centers. *Clinical Orthopaedics and Related Research, 157*, 64, 69.

Craxford, A. D., Stevens, J., & Park, C. (1982). Management of the deformed rheumatoid forefoot: A comparison of conservative and surgical methods. *Clinical Orthopaedics and Related Research, 166*, 121–126.

Daly, P. J., & Johnson, K. A. (1992). Treatment of painful subluxation or dislocation at the second and third metatarsophalangeal joints by partial proxial phalanx excision and subtotal webbing. *Clinical Orthopaedics and Related Research, 278*, 164–170.

Dedrich, D. K., McCune, W. S., & Smith, W. S. (1990). Rheumatoid arthritis presenting as spreading of the toes. *Journal of Bone and Joint Surgery, 72A*, 463–464.

Downey, D. J., Simkin, P. A., Mack, L. A., Richardson, M. L., Kilcoyne, R. F., & Hansen, S. T. (1988). Tibialis posterior tendon rupture: A cause of rheumatoid flat foot. *Arthritis and Rheumatism, 31*(3), 441–446.

Elbar, J. E., Thomas, W. K., Weinfeld, M. S., & Potter, T. A. (1976). Talonavicular arthrodesis for rheumatoid arthritis of the hindfoot. *Orthopedic Clinics of North America, 7*(4), 821–826.

Faithful, D. K., & Savill, D. L. (1971). Review of the results of excision of metatarsal heads in patients with rheumatoid arthritis. *Annals of Rheumatic Disease, 30*, 201–202.

Feiwell, L. A., & Cracchiolo, A. (1994). The use of internal fixation in performing triple arthrodesis in adults. *The Foot, 4*, 10–14.

Figgie, H. E. III, Unger, A. S., Inglis, A. E., Kraay, M. J., & Figgie, M. P. (1991). Total ankle arthroplasty. In W. Petty (Ed.), *Total joint replacement* (pp. 749–760). Philadelphia: Saunders.

Figgie, M. P., O'Malley, M. J., Ranawat, C., Inglis, A. E., & Sculco, T. P. (1993). Triple arthrodesis in rheumatoid arthritis. *Clinical Orthopaedics and Related Research, 292*, 250–254.

Friscia, D. A. (1996). Subtalar fusion. In G. B. Pfeefer, & C. C. Frey (Eds.), *Current practices in foot and ankle surgery* (pp. 157–172). New York: McGraw-Hill.

Gainor, B. J., Epstein, R. G., Henstorf, J. E., & Olson, S. (1988). Metatarsal head resection for rheumatoid deformities of the forefoot. *Clinical Orthopaedics and Related Research, 230*, 207–213.

Hassalo, L. G., Wilkens, R. F., Toomey, H. E., Darges, D. E., & Hansen, S. T. (1987). Forefoot surgery in rheumatoid arthritis: Subjective assessment of outcomes. *Foot and Ankle, 8,* 148–151.

Hughes, J., Grace, D., Clark, P., & Klenerman, L. (1991). Metatarsal head excision for rheumatoid arthritis: Four-year follow-up of 68 feet with and without hallux fusion. *Acta Orthopaedica Scandinavica, 62,* 63–66.

Janisse, D. J. (1995a). Pedorthics and the podiatrist. *Podiatry Today, 7,* 29–32.

Janisse, D. J. (1995b). Prescription insoles and footwear. *Clinics in Podiatric Medicine and Surgery, 12,* 41–61.

Janisse, D. J. (1995c). The shoe in rehabilitation of the foot and ankle. In G. J. Sammarco (Ed.), *Rehabilitation of the foot and ankle* (pp. 339–349). St. Louis, MO: Mosby-Year Book.

Janisse, D. J. (1995d). Pedorthics in rehabilitation of the foot and ankle. In G. J. Sammarco (Ed.), *Rehabilitation of the foot and ankle* (pp. 351–364). St. Louis, MO: Mosby-Year Book.

Johnson, K. A. (1994). Cheveron osteotomy. In K. A. Johnson (Ed.), *Master techniques in orthopedics: The foot and ankle* (pp. 31–48). New York: Raven Press.

Kates, A., Kessel, L., & Kay, A. (1967). Arthroplasty of the forefoot. *Journal of Bone and Joint Surgery, 49B,* 552–557.

King, H. A., Watkins, T. B., & Samuelson, K. M. (1980). Analysis of foot position in ankle arthrodesis and its influence in gait. *Foot and Ankle, 1,* 44–49.

Kitaoka, H. B., & Johnson, K. A. (1996). Total ankle arthroplasty. In B. F. Morrey (Ed.), *Reconstructive surgery of the joints* (pp. 1757–1770). New York: Churchill Livingstone.

Lipscomb, P. R., Benson, G. M., & Sones, D. A. (1972). Resection of proximal phalanges and metatarsal condyles for deformities of the forefoot due to rheumatoid arthritis. *Clinical Orthopaedics and Related Research, 82,* 24–31.

Mann, R. A., & Thompson, F. M. (1984). Arthrodesis of the first metatarsophalaneal joint for hallux valgus in rheumatoid arthritis. *Journal of Bone and Joint Surgery, 66A,* 687–692.

McGarvey, S. R., & Johnson, K. A. (1988). Keller arthroplasty in combination with resection arthroplasty of the lesser metatarsophalangeal joints in rheumatoid arthritis. *Foot and Ankle, 9,* 75–80.

Michelson, J., Easley, M., Wigley, F. M., & Hellmann, D. (1995). Posterior tibial tendon dysfunction in rheumatoid arthritis. *Foot and Ankle, 16,* 156–161.

Moeckel, B. H., Sculco, T. P., Alexiades, M. M., Dossick, P. H., Inglis, A. E., & Ranawat, C. S. (1992). The double-stem silicone-rubber implant for rheumatoid arthritis of the first metatarsophalangeal joint: Long term results. *Journal of Bone and Joint Surgery, 74A,* 564–570.

Morgan, C. D., Henke, J. A., Bailey, R. W., & Kaufer, H. (1985). Long term results of tibiotalar arthrodesis. *Journal of Bone and Joint Surgery, 67A,* 546.

Newman, R. J., & Fitton, J. M. (1983). Conservation of metatarsal head in surgery of rheumatoid arthritis of the forefoot. *Acta Orthopaedica Scandinavica, 54,* 417–421.

Pincus, T., & Callahan, L. F. (1992). Rheumatology function tests: Grip strength, walking time, button test and questionnaires document and predict long-term morbidity and mortality in rheumatoid arthritis. *Journal of Rheumatology, 19,* 1051–1057.

Roth, R. D. (1986). The role of the podiatrist in the rheumatology team. In G. Ehrlich (Ed.), *Rehabilitation management of rheumatic conditions* (pp. 286–289). Baltimore: Williams & Wilkins.

Russotti, G. J., Johnson, K. A., & Cass, J. R. (1988). Tibiocalcaneal arthrodesis for arthritis of the hind part of the foot. *Journal of Bone and Joint Surgery, 70A,* 1304–1307.

Saltman, C. L. (1996). Rheumatoid forefoot reconstruction. In B. F. Morrey (Ed.), *Reconstructive surgery of the joints* (pp. 197–212). New York: Churchill Livingstone.

Sebold, E. J., & Cracchiolo, A. (1996). The use of titanium grommets in silicone implant arthroplasty of the hallux metatarsophalangeal joint. *Foot and Ankle, 17,* 145–151.

Shephard, E. (1975). Intermetarso-phalangeal bursitis in the causation of Morton's metatarsalgia. *Journal of Bone and Joint Surgery, 57B,* 115–116.

Spiegel, T. M., & Spiegel, J. S. (1982). Rheumatoid arthritis in the foot and ankle: Diagnosis, pathology, and treatment. *Foot and Ankle, 2,* 318–324.

Stockey, I., Betts, R. P., Eng, C., Getty, C. J. M., Rowley, D. I., & Duckworth, T. (1989). A prospective study of forefoot arthroplasty. *Clinical Orthopaedics and Related Research, 248,* 213–218.

Swanson, A. B., deGroot Swanson, G., Maupin, B. K., Shi, S., Petrus, J. G., Alander, D. H., & Cesrani, V. A. (1991). The use of a grommet bone liner for flexible hinge implant arthroplasty of the great toe. *Foot and Ankle, 12,* 149–155.

Vahvanen, V., Pirainen, H., & Kettunen, P. (1980). Resection arthroplasty of the metatarsophalangeal joints in rheumatoid arthritis: A follow-up study of 100 patients. *Scandinavian Journal of Rheumatology, 9,* 257–265.

Watson, M. S. (1974). A long-term follow-up of forefoot arthroplasty. *Journal of Bone and Joint Surgery, 56B,* 527–533.

Appendix 1

Foot Function Index

Name: _____ ID: _____ Date: ___/___/___ Total Score: _____

ACTIVITY LIMITATION

The line next to each item represents how often you did something in the past week. On the far left is "None of the time" and on the far right is "All of the time". Place a mark on the line to indicate how often you performed the following activities in the past week because of your *feet*. Mark NA on the line to the far right of the item if you did not perform this activity during the *past week*.

EXAMPLE: How much of the time did you:

0. Wear shoes when walking in the house? . . . . None of the time _____ All of the time

A. HOW MUCH OF THE TIME DID YOU:

1. Use a cane, crutches or a walker indoors? . . . . None of the time _____ All of the time
2. Use a cane, crutches or a walker outdoors? . . . . None of the time _____ All of the time
3. Stay indoors most of the day because of foot problems?
4. Stay in bed most of the day because of foot problems? . . . . None of the time _____ All of the time
5. Limit your activities because of foot problems? . . . . None of the time _____ All of the time

PAIN

The line next to each item represents the amount of pain you typically had in each situation. On the far left is "No pain" and on the far right is "The worst pain imaginable". Place a mark on the line to indicate how bad your *foot* pain was in each of the following situations during the past week. If you were not involved in one or more of these situations, mark that item NA.

B. HOW SEVERE WAS YOUR *FOOT* PAIN: NA

1. At its worst? . . . . No pain _____ Worst pain imaginable _____
2. Before you get up in the morning? . . . . No pain _____ Worst pain imaginable _____
3. When you walked barefoot? . . . . No pain _____ Worst pain imaginable _____
4. When you stood barefoot? . . . . No pain _____ Worst pain imaginable _____
5. When you walked wearing shoes? . . . . No pain _____ Worst pain imaginable _____
6. When you stood wearing shoes? . . . . No pain _____ Worst pain imaginable _____
7. When you walked wearing orthotics? . . . . No pain _____ Worst pain imaginable _____
8. When you stood wearing orthotics? . . . . No pain _____ Worst pain imaginable _____
9. At the end of the day? . . . . No pain _____ Worst pain imaginable _____

Appendix 1 (cont.)

DISABILITY

The line next to each item represents the amount of difficulty you had performing an activity. On the far left is "No Difficulty" and on the far right is "So difficult unable". Place a mark on the line to indicate how much difficulty you had performing each activity because of your *feet* during the past week. If you did not perform an activity during the past week, mark that item NA.

C. HOW MUCH DIFFICULTY DID YOU HAVE: NA

1. Walking around the house? .... No difficulty _____ So difficult unable _____
2. Walking outside on uneven ground? .... No difficulty _____ So difficult unable _____
3. Walking four or more blocks? .... No difficulty _____ So difficult unable _____
4. Climbing stairs? .... No difficulty _____ So difficult unable _____
5. Descending stairs? .... No difficulty _____ So difficult unable _____
6. Standing on tip toes? .... No difficulty _____ So difficult unable _____
7. Getting out of a chair? .... No difficulty _____ So difficult unable _____
8. Climbing up or down curbs? .... No difficulty _____ So difficult unable _____
9. Walking fast or running? .... No difficulty _____ So difficult unable _____

_____ / _____ — _____ %

Note. Copyright by Elly Budiman-Mak. Reprinted with permission. This work was supported by the Midwest Center for Health Services and Policy Research, Veterans Affairs Hines Hospital, and grant support from the Department of Veterans Affairs. When reproducing this form to normal size, each line between "None of the time" and "All of the time" should be 10 cm long.

Appendix 2
Foot Rules To Live By

1. Check your feet often. They are critical to your ability to remain mobile.
2. Inspect your toes and the space between them daily for blisters, cuts, and scratches.
3. Inspect your feet for red areas indicating pressure on both the tops of your toes and the sides and bottoms of your feet. Using a hand mirror can help.
4. Wash your feet daily and dry carefully, especially between the toes.
5. Avoid using chemical agents to remove corns and calluses.
6. Cut toe nails straight across.
7. Wear properly fitted stockings (wrinkles can cause pressure areas; tight socks can squeeze toes).
8. Avoid wearing elastic garters or other tight-fitting bands around your legs.
9. Arthritis can cause the position of the bones in your feet to change. You may have to modify your footwear often.
10. Shoes should be comfortable at the time of purchase. Do not depend on them to stretch with wear.
11. Proper fit is important. There should be adequate width and depth to avoid pressure on the toes. The back of the shoe should be snug around your heel.
12. You should seek the advice of a professional with expertise in foot care when:
    • all shoes cause you pain;
    • you feel like you are walking on marbles;
    • shoes cause painful pressure areas on your toes or feet;
    • your ankles turn in, or you wear out the soles of your shoes unevenly.

Note. From "Care of the Arthritis Foot" brochure, by P. W. Minor and Son Shoe Company. Reprinted with permission.

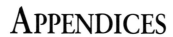

APPENDICES

Appendix A
Classification of Rheumatoid Arthritis

Stage I, Early

* 1. No destructive changes on roentgenographic examination

2. Radiographic evidence of osteoporosis may be present

Stage II, Moderate

* 1. Radiographic evidence of osteoporosis, with or without slight subchondral bone destruction; slight cartilage destruction may be present

* 2. No joint deformities, although limitation of joint mobility may be present

3. Adjacent muscle atrophy

4. Extraarticular soft tissue lesions, such as nodules and tenosynovitis may be present

Stage III, Severe

* 1. Radiographic evidence of cartilage and bone destruction, in addition to osteoporosis

* 2. Joint deformity, such as subluxation; ulnar deviation, or hyperextension, without fibrous or bony ankylosis

3. Extensive muscle atrophy

4. Extraarticular soft tissue lesions, such as nodules and tenosynovitis may be present

Stage IV, Terminal

* 1. Fibrous or bony ankylosis

2. Criteria of stage III

*The criteria prefaced by an asterisk are those that must be present to permit classification of a patient in any particular stage or grade. From Steinbrocker O., Traeger CH, Batterman RC: Therapeutic criteria in rheumatoid arthritis. *Journal of the American Medical Association, 140,* 659–652, 1949, with permission.

Appendix B
Criteria for Classification of Functional Status in Rheumatoid Arthritis*

Class I: Completely able to perform usual activities of daily living (self-care, vocational, and avocational)

Class II: Able to perform usual self-care and vocational activities, but limited in avocational activities

Class III: Able to perform usual self-care activities, but limited in vocational and avocational activities

Class IV: Limited in ability to perform usual self-care, vocational, and avocational activities

---

*Usual self-care activities include dressing, feeding, bathing, grooming, and toileting. Avocational (recreational and/or leisure) and vocational (work, school, homemaking) activities are patient-desired and age- and sex-specific. From Hochberg, MC, Chang, RW, Dwosh I, et al: The American College of Rheumatology 1991 revised criteria for the classification of global functional status in rheumatoid arthritis. *Arthritis and Rheumatology 35,* 498–502, 1992, with permission from Lippincott-Raven Publishers.

Appendix C
SF-36 Health Survey

INSTRUCTIONS: This survey asks for your views about your health. This information will help keep track of how you feel and how well you are able to do your usual activities.

Answer every question by marking the answer as indicated. If you are unsure about how to answer a question, please give the best answer you can.

1. In general, would you say your health is:

(circle one)

Q100   Excellent 1
         Very good 2
         Good 3
         Fair 4
         Poor 5

2. *Compared to one year ago,* how would you rate your health in general *now?*

(circle one)

Q101   Much better now than one year ago 1
         Somewhat better now than one year ago 2
         About the same as one year ago 3
         Somewhat worse now than one year ago 4
         Much worse now than one year ago 5

3. The following items are about activities you might do during a typical day. does *your health now limit you* in these activities? If so, how much?

(circle one number on each line)

ACTIVITIES		Yes, Limited A Lot	Yes, Limited A Little	No, Not Limited At All
a. **Vigorous activities**, such as running, lifting heavy objects, participating in strenuous sports	Q102	1	2	3
b. **Moderate activities**, such as moving a table, pushing a vacuum cleaner, bowling, or playing golf	Q103	1	2	3
c. Lifting or carrying groceries	Q104	1	2	3
d. Climbing **several** flights of stairs	Q105	1	2	3
e. Climbing **one** flight of stairs	Q106	1	2	3
f. Bending, kneeling, or stooping	Q107	1	2	3
g. Walking **more than a mile**	Q108	1	2	3
h. Walking **several blocks**	Q109	1	2	3
i. Walking **one block**	Q110	1	2	3
j. Bathing or dressing yourself	Q111	1	2	3

Appendix C (cont.)

4. During the *past 4 weeks* have you had any of the following problems with your work or other regular daily activities *as a result of your physical health*

		(circle one number on each line)	
		YES	**NO**
a. Cut down on the amount of time you spent on work or other activities	Q113	1	2
b. **Accomplished less** than you would like	Q113	1	2
c. Were limited in the **kind** of work or other activities	Q114	1	2
d. Had **difficulty** performing the work or other activities (for example, it took extra effort)	Q115	1	2

5. During the *past 4 weeks* have you had any of the following problems with your work or other regular daily activities *as a result of your any emotional problems* (such as feeling depressed or anxious)?

		(circle one number on each line)	
		YES	**NO**
a. Cut down the **amount of time you spent on work or other activities**	Q116	1	2
b. **Accomplished less** than you would like	Q117	1	2
c. Didn't do work or other activities as **carefully as usual**	Q118	1	2

6. During the *past 4 weeks,* to what extent has your physical health or emotional problems interfered with your normal social activities with family, friends, neighbors, or groups?

(circle one)

Q119
Not at all 1
Slightly 2
Moderately 3
Quite a bit 4
Extremely 5

7. How much *bodily* pain have you had during the *past 4 weeks?*

(circle one)

Q120
None 1
Very mild 2
Mild 3
Moderate 4
Severe 5
Very severe 6

Appendix C (cont.)

8. During the *past 4 weeks* how much did *pain* interfere with your normal work (including both work outside the home and housework)?

(circle one)

Q121   Not at all 1
        A little bit 2
        Moderately 3
        Quite a bit 4
        Extremely 5

9. These questions are about how you feel and how things have been with you **during the past 4 weeks**. For each question, please give the one answer that comes closest to the way you have been feeling. How much of the time during the **past 4 weeks—**

(circle one number on each line)

		All of the Time	Most of the Time	A Good Bit of the Time	Some of the Time	A Little of the Time	None of the Time
a. Did you feel full of pep?	Q122	1	2	3	4	5	6
b. Have you been a very nervous person?	Q123	1	2	3	4	5	6
c. Have you felt so down in the dumps that nothing could cheer you up?	Q124	1	2	3	4	5	6
d. Have you felt calm and peaceful?	Q125	1	2	3	4	5	6
e. Did you have a lot of energy?	Q126	1	2	3	4	5	6
f. Have you felt downhearted and blue?	Q127	1	2	3	4	5	6
g. Did you feel worn out?	Q128	1	2	3	4	5	6
h. Have you been a happy person?	Q129	1	2	3	4	5	6
i. Did you feel tired?	Q130	1	2	3	4	5	6

10. During the *past 4 weeks,* how much of the time has your *physical health or emotional problems* interfered with your social activities (like visiting with friends, relatives, etc.)?

(circle one)

Q131   All of the time 1
        Most of the time 2
        Some of the time 3
        A little of the time 4
        None of the time 5

11. How TRUE or FALSE is *each* of the following statements for you?

(circle one number on each line)

		Definitely True	Mostly True	Don't Know	Mostly False	Definitely False
a. I seem to get sick a little easier than other people	Q132	1	2	3	4	5
b. I am as healthy as anybody I know	Q133	1	2	3	4	5
c. I expect my health to get worse	Q134	1	2	3	4	5
d. My health is excellent	Q135	1	2	3	4	5

Appendix D
Resources

Organization Resources

THE ARTHRITIS FOUNDATION
1330 W. Peachtree Street
Atlanta, GA 30309
404–872–7100   1–800–283–7800
www.arthritis.org

Provides an excellent booklet on each of the rheumatic diseases, self-management techniques and on specific medications at no charge. They also have several excellent books on managing arthritis.

Aquatic and land-based exercise classses and the Arthritis Self-Management Course nationwide.

Some chapters offer a free health video lending library. They can refer patients to rheumatologists.

THE ARTHRITIS SOCIETY
National Office
250 Bloor Street East, Suite 901
Toronto, ON M4W 3P2
Phone: 416–967–1414
Fax: 416–967–7171

Internet Address: *www.arthritis.ca*

Offers: specialized patient-care programs, recreational exercise programs, resource libraries and consumer education material.

Internet Resources

Searching "arthritis" on the Internet brings up an extensive array of resources and sales pitches, unproven remedies, and misinformation (11,262 listings), "HOTBOT" is one of the best search directories for information on diseases.

1. Arthritis Foundation and The Arthritis Society, see addresses above.

2. The Amazon Bookstore (amazon.com) is the easiest online bookseller to search. There are about 5 current self-help books on OA.

3. Abledata is a National database on adaptive equipment and assistive devices. (*www.abledata.com*)

4. One Step Ahead News, *www.osanews.com*–The Web's online news magazine for people with disabilities, provides excellent links to other sites related to coping with disabilities including one on Americans with Disabilities Act (*www.osanews.com/Links/ada.htm*)

5. Minnesota Mining Company, Guide to arthritis (*http://arthritis.miningaco.com/msub7.htm*) Excellent resources and information.

INDEX

Surgical Rehabilitation Index